Framing ADHD Children

Framing ADHD Children

*A Critical Examination of
the History, Discourse,
and Everyday Experience of
Attention Deficit/Hyperactivity
Disorder*

Adam Rafalovich

LEXINGTON BOOKS
Lanham • Boulder • New York • Toronto • Oxford

KH

To protect the anonymity of individuals who were interviewed, real names have not been used.

LEXINGTON BOOKS

Published in the United States of America
by Lexington Books
An imprint of The Rowman & Littlefield Publishing Group, Inc.
4501 Forbes Boulevard, Suite 200, Lanham, Maryland 20706

PO Box 317
Oxford
OX2 9RU, UK

British Library Cataloguing in Publication Information Available

Library of Congress Cataloging-in-Publication Data

Rafalovich, Adam, 1970–
  Framing ADHD children : a critical examination of the history, discourse, and everyday experience of attention deficit/hyperactivity disorder / Adam Rafalovich.
      p. cm.
  Includes bibliographical references and index.
  ISBN 0-7391-0747-X (cloth : alk. paper)
  1. Attention-deficit hyperactivity disorder. I. Title.
RJ506.H9R34 2004
616.85'89—dc22   2004003005

Printed in the United States of America

♾™ The paper used in this publication meets the minimum requirements of American National Standard for Information Sciences—Permanence of Paper for Printed Library Materials, ANSI/NISO Z39.48–1992.

8/21/05

In loving memory of Derrick G., the "goat" of Clear Creek

Contents

Acknowledgments   ix

1   Introduction   1

2   Before We Called It ADHD: Idiocy, Imbecility, and *Encephalitis Lethargica*   21

3   Psychodynamic versus Neurological ADHD Narratives: Clinicians Discuss *DSM IV* and the Essences of ADHD   35

4   Clinicians as the Mediators of ADHD Suspicion and Treatment   63

5   The Realm of Semiformal Suspicion: Framing ADHD in the Classroom   89

6   Responding to ADHD: School Curricula, Simplified Assignments, and Gender   109

7   Parents' Accounts: How Trouble Becomes ADHD   129

8   Developing Informal Expertise: How Parents Negotiate the Meaning of ADHD   151

9   Conclusion   177

Bibliography   183

Index   193

About the Author   197

Acknowledgments

Writing this book has introduced me to the truth of this maxim: apart we cannot, together we can. Being the author by no means designates me as the sole contributor to the contents of these pages. Through their participation in my research, their willingness to read countless drafts of this manuscript, and the passion they inspire in me, numerous people have made this book possible.

I would first like to thank all of the people who participated as interview respondents for this project. Their stories are the basis of this book, and they do much to show the human side of ADHD. Thank you for all that you have taught me about myself and about the world.

Special consideration must be given to Bob Ratner, professor emeritus of sociology at the University of British Columbia (UBC), without whom this project would have never begun, nor would it have ever finished. Through his example, Professor Ratner has taught me the value of being a good and thorough researcher, but more importantly, how to be a member of the intellectual community. His help with my writing and analytical skills has provided the foundation for what I hope will be a promising academic career. Special thanks also go out to Thomas Kemple and Janice Graham of UBC, who took much care in helping me improve numerous areas of this study; Karen Pugliesi of Northern Arizona University, who introduced me to the sociology of mental health ten years ago; the wonderful staff at the University of California at San Francisco, and UBC medical libraries; Jon R. Dowd for all of the brilliance over the years; Chase Browning for being one of the smartest people alive; Brady E. Moss for letting me know that idiocy is truly a political phenomenon; Kim Sherrell for the endless hours of theoretical discussion that made this analysis richer and better; Dean K. Ledbetter and Doug Striley for showing me what a *real* work ethic is about; my colleagues at Texas Tech University for all of the support in getting this project completed; and finally, that kid in the park, whose name I'll never know, who ran by me and shouted "I'm ADHD!" and started my mind thinking about this project.

I want to finally mention the person who makes the foundation of my life possible: my wife, and life partner, Nell. She has taught me the true value of friendship, giving unyielding support in my times of triumph and self-doubt. The perseverance that has enabled this book comes from you as much as it does from me. This is ours.

Chapter One

Introduction

Attention Deficit-Hyperactivity Disorder (American Psychiatric Association 1994, 83-85), also known as ADHD, or more colloquially as ADD, is a mental disorder and an acronym that is seemingly embedded in North American consciousness. The portrayals of persons with ADHD in our popular culture illustrate how widely recognized this disorder has become. A recent example can be seen in the James Foley film *Confidence* (2002), featuring Dustin Hoffman as Winston King, a gum-chewing, pill-popping, "severely ADD" con artist. At one point King is admonished by his fellow grifter and nemesis, Jake (played by Edward Burns), to "Get the ADD under control." As the plot unfolds, it is obvious that King will never rein in his neurological malfunctions. In fact, it is the condition of ADHD that adds to King's intrigue, enhancing his volatility, establishing his character as a gangster, a social misfit. His behavior becomes increasingly erratic, prompting the declaration in one of his more violent moments that he is "impulsive." As much as it draws the audience to Hoffman's character, this impulsiveness is presented as a disadvantage for King, contributing to his being deceived by Jake and his capture by the authorities. As impulsiveness has come to symbolize incompetence and disability in our society, Jake, in the many ways he methodically manipulates King, has a distinct and unfair psychological advantage over him.

The basic symptoms of ADHD can be summarized by anyone who reads a newspaper, watches the news, or participates in public discourse to any degree. Virtually everyone I speak with about ADHD has an opinion regarding the disorder, and on discovering my sociological interest in the topic, people readily ask my opinions: Is ADHD real? Is Ritalin prescribed too frequently? How can you tell if ADHD exists? Does someone outgrow ADHD? Is ADHD really a symptom of bad parenting? of bad schools? Questions such as these continue ad infinitum. In addressing them over the years, and in doing the research necessary for the writing of this book, I have become acutely aware of how vast and varied the many answers to them are. Indeed, medical science is no longer the sole proprietor of ADHD discourse, nor is any one perspective, for that matter. Our contemporary discussion of ADHD is represented by a plurality of views: academic, clinical, pop cultural, journalistic, and so on. The various and pluralized interpretations of what does or does not constitute ADHD that comprise the motley tapestry of today's ADHD discourse are largely a product of the vagaries of this disorder. People easily join the ADHD discussion because they can relate to it. The basic "symptoms" of ADHD summarize what most Western humans have experienced at one time or another: impulsivity, distractibility, task incompletion—do these not encapsulate many of our experiences in modern life?

The vagueness of what constitutes ADHD has undoubtedly contributed to the vast number of children who are today diagnosed with the disorder. According to the American Academy of Pediatrics, just under four million schoolchildren in the United States have been diagnosed with some form of ADHD, two million of whom are taking Ritalin; numerous others take another stimulant medication, such as Adderall, Dexedrine, or Cylert. Moreover, since 1985, the prevalence rate for Ritalin prescriptions in the United States has increased 327 percent (Lipman 2002). At the same time, we live in an era in which psychotherapy as a treatment option for problem children is practically non-existent (Walker 1998). Despite opinions of the many clinicians, social scientists, and cultural critics who contend that the ADHD diagnosis is replete with reliability and validity issues, the disorder is regarded as a significant medical problem.

The fact that ADHD *is* a medical problem is the sole underpinning of this book. Being a sociologist, I almost instinctively adopt the stance that the criteria describing mental disorders are intertwined with a variety of social forces. As sociology is implicitly skeptical toward strictly biochemical definitions of mental health, the job of this book is to explore how social forces bear on the medical problem of ADHD. In examining these forces, I draw upon two divergent yet useful perspectives. The first perspective from which I examine ADHD stems from the sociological study of how deviant behavior becomes "medicalized" or perceived to be a medical problem. The second perspective is "genealogical," emphasizing the role played by historical and contemporary discourses about ADHD in shaping people's everyday conceptions of the disorder. In demonstrating this relationship between discourse and everyday experience, and in demonstrating how ADHD is medicalized, this book is centered on intensive interviews with the people most involved with ADHD, including clinicians, teachers, parents, and, to a lesser extent, ADHD children. For the remainder of this section of the introduction I will summarize aspects of both of these perspectives and highlight why unifying them is important in the ongoing social study of ADHD.

Acknowledging Peter Conrad

Exemplifying a critical sociological perspective on ADHD, and providing much reason to be skeptical of the medical legitimacy of today's ADHD epidemic, is the work of Peter Conrad (1975, 1976; Conrad and Potter 2000). Conrad's (1975, 1976) analyses of ADHD invoke sociological discussions of mental deviance, specifically models that explain how socially inappropriate or antagonistic behavior are defined through medical labels. His groundbreaking *Identifying Hyperactive Children* (1976), the "first empirical analysis of the process of medicalization," (5) examines how medical professionals construct the problem of hyperkinesis[1] from deviant childhood behavior. Conrad's analysis rests upon an interest in the growing influence of medical practice in social life:

> What is significant . . . is the expansion of the sphere where medicine now functions as an agent of social control. In the wake of a general humanitarian trend, the success and prestige of modern medicine, the increasing acceptance of deterministic social and medical concepts, the technological growth of the twentieth century and the diminution of religion as a viable institution of control, more and more deviant behavior has come into the province of medicine (4-5).

Drawing from a variety of sources, Conrad (1976, 12) argues that the conversion of unconventional childhood behavior into the medical entity of hyperkinesis can be traced to the interplay among three agents: "(1) the pharmaceutical revolution, (2) trends in the medical profession, and (3) government action." Conrad's "pharmaceutical revolution" analysis points the finger at the party responsible for the synthesis and marketing of Ritalin, Ciba (Ritalin is now marketed and distributed by Novartis Pharmaceuticals), which in the 1960s began a large-scale advertising campaign that targeted both medical and educational sectors of American society. Conrad's examination of medical trends refers to the increased interpretation of behavioral problems as biochemical or organic in origin. The "government action" facet of Conrad's analysis directs attention at government agencies, in this case the U.S. Public Health Service, which were responsible for unifying the symptoms of hyperkinesis into the clinical entity of "minimal brain dysfunction," or MBD.

This three fold description of the agents that contributed to the discovery of the hyperkinesis phenomenon argues that the public and institutional definition of hyperkinesis is largely influenced by actions taken by these agents. From Conrad's perspective, these three entities reflect the sizable disparity in power between lay actors and formal organizations. The invention of hyperkinesis and the terms MBD and, later, ADHD denote intensified "expert control," in which the use of obscure and inaccessible language alienate lay persons from the discussion. As Conrad (1975) states: "By defining a problem as medical it [*sic*] is removed from the public realm where there can be discussion by ordinary people and put on a plane where only medical people can discuss it" (Conrad 1975, 18). Problems defined as medical rather than "ordinary" produce a daunting chasm of knowledge between those who explain the problem of hyperkinesis and their audience. Borrowing from Howard S. Becker, Conrad (1976, 15) argues that this chasm was begun by "moral entrepreneurs"—agents who bring attention to a problem in society they believe to be of particular concern and, in drawing this attention, begin the organizational response to behaviors deemed to be deviant. Through describing a combination of the formal nomenclature of modern medicine and the passionate voice of moral entrepreneurs, Conrad sets the stage for an important empirical contribution to "classic" deviance theory.

Many of the assertions posited by Conrad and others conceptualize knowledge systems as originating in the expert arena and disseminating to the public. As modern medicine, for example, accumulates one form of knowledge, it becomes a resource for the segments of society that need and want to know more about medical problems. Within this asymmetrical knowledge relationship, many argue, is the potential for the abuse of power, perhaps through the literal fabrication of social problems. Conrad contends that the medical realm, for example, is where ADHD had effectively originated and is—through medicine's own invention—the location of the solution for ADHD. The medical realm, in this instance, invents (or "socially constructs," in sociological terms) a problem and then claims ownership of the feasible measures for rectifying it. As the problem and solution become more known, and hence more legitimate, the knowledge asymmetry between medical and lay realms is maintained and exacerbated. Such inequity fosters a dependency in which the public continually seeks medical professionals for the definition of problems outside of the lay purview.

Many of the sociological interpretations of mental illness that influence Conrad's early work and my perspectives in this book are derived from Symbolic Interactionism—a perspective in sociology that postulates that human life becomes meaningful through social interactions that are founded upon shared symbolic frameworks (Blumer 1969). Jack Douglas (1970, vii) provides a summary of some of the tenets of this perspective:

> Human social order is necessarily problematic. Since we must have social order to exist, but cannot achieve it by simply living naturally, it becomes a crucial problem of our existence which we must solve if we are to exist at all.
>
> Man is also necessarily a symbolic animal, for it is only his capacity to create and work with symbols which he takes in some way to be real that allows him to solve the necessary problem of social order. Being unable to rely on shared instincts (or shared imprintings) to coordinate his interactions with his fellows, man must substitute a shared universe of (symbolic) meanings to achieve that coordination.

Implied here is the notion that human societies are based upon shared interpretations of the world. Humans act according to a symbolic order, constituting the stability of social life, which sociologists can analyze on many different levels: interpersonal, institutional, cultural, and so on. As they apply to the study of deviant behavior, Symbolic Interactionist stances are often concerned with the mechanisms that deploy a particular symbolic device and infuse an ideology into the public. Conrad's (1975, 1976) content analysis of hyperactivity, for example, measures the symbolic power of the pharmaceutical industry by counting the number of advertisements in medical journals which such companies use to sway clinical practices. Attached to the analysis of this deployment of symbols is an examination of the power relations associated with them. It is fitting, then, that sociologists often position themselves as advocates for those who become objectified or dehumanized by such a symbolic order. Such advocacy often prompts poignant critique of the origins of symbolic power.

Predominant theoretical positions in the sociology of mental illness are characterized by a duality, which places the "informal" or everyday realm against the "formal" or medicalizing realm (Emerson and Messinger 1977; Goffman 1961). Previous studies have asserted that medicalization shifts interpretations of deviant behavior from seeing such behavior as "bad" to seeing it as "sick" (Conrad and Schneider 1980). The informal realm provides "cultural scripts" for personal conduct, defining normal or abnormal behavior within a given social context. The formal realm, on the other hand, is inextricably linked to institutions and is the place of official mental disorder diagnoses. The formal realm has a profound interdependence with the informal. For example, Scheff (1999) contends that behaviors become formally described as states of mental illness when "residual rules" are consistently broken in the informal context. Violation of these rules is not necessarily defined as criminal or impolite; these violations denote something that "just isn't quite right" with the individual. It is argued that modern psychiatry exploits these ambiguities in the informal realm and applies medical labels that offer technical explanations for previously inexplicable behavior. Mental disorder, it is argued, is a phenomenon whose etiology can be discussed through an examination of cultural and institutional antecedents rather than psychological or physiological ones (Grusky and Pollner 1981). From the perspective of the formal institutional realm, the informal label of "weirdo" represents a misunderstood phenomenon. He/she may not be "weird" but perhaps "hebephrenic," "bi-polar," or "ADHD."

These tenets of the sociology of mental health have been very influential in the conceptualization and writing of this book. As subsequent chapters illustrate, the everyday experiences of ADHD are characterized by marked knowledge imbalances between lay actors and medical practitioners—discrepancies that invariably influence the way ADHD is understood, suspected, diagnosed, and treated. Further, this discrepancy in knowledge illustrates the tremendous power the formal realm holds over the informal. What is important to add to such perspectives are explorations of how the often contradictory discussions about ADHD influence the ways everyday people negotiate what constitutes ADHD, and what, if anything, are its appropriate lines of treatment. Even though aspects of ADHD knowledge are disseminated unilaterally, people may assert a tremendous amount of agency in how they interpret the disorder. As this book demonstrates, "freedom of choice" in interpreting ADHD is not exercised just by concerned parents, but by all of the different groups of people I interviewed. There is, therefore, another variable that influences people's perceptions of ADHD, enabling them to confirm, or to doubt, the disorder's validity.

Approaches to Genealogical Understandings of ADHD

Its various interpretations demonstrate that ADHD is far from being unified by an all-encompassing discourse. Because of this, the historical and contemporary discourses that have constituted previous and present notions about ADHD require meticulous scholarly treatment. In undertaking this treatment, the present book attempts to either break from or further some of the aforementioned perspectives in the sociology of mental health. Through discussing interviews with persons most closely associated with ADHD in conjunction with analyses of the detailed historical and contemporary discourses that provide the "understanding" of the disorder, this study will demonstrate how the variety of ADHD discussions found in medical journals, mental health manuals, and popular reading influence and are influenced by people's everyday experiences. Prior to describing the people I interviewed for this book, allow me to briefly explain what is known as the "genealogical approach" to mental disorder and why it is relevant for a social understanding of ADHD.

A genealogical analysis may begin by articulating ADHD as a collection of historically contingent concepts and statements which do not necessarily adhere to one discipline or institutional context and cannot be perfectly traceable to any specific social agent. As the "social product" of discursive formations, diagnoses of ADHD and other mental disorders are always in a state of flux, always contested and contestable. This condition is demonstrated by the many symptoms and namesakes ADHD has owned over the last century and also by the unclear epidemiology of the disorder.

Since the early 1900s ADHD-like symptoms have included, but are certainly not limited to (1) poor performance in school; (2) extreme extroversion; (3) outbursts of violent behavior; (4) inability to "stay on task"; (5) thievery; (6) disturbances in sleep patterns; (7) morality inconsistent with age; and (8) forgetfulness. Some of these may or may not seem related to today's conceptions of ADHD, and yet these symptoms are historically linked to today's clinical interpretations of this disorder. All of these symptoms and many more have comprised a variety of diagnoses over the years, depending upon historical period. Some of these previous ADHD disease names include: (1) *encephalitis lethargica* (sequelae of); (2) minimal brain damage; (3) minimal cerebral palsy; (4) mild retardation; (5) minimal brain dysfunction; (6) hyperkinesis; and (7) atypical ego development. Although these categories represent many historical antecedents of today's discussion of ADHD, they should not be considered entirely interchangeable; however, they all address the problems of childhood that ultimately crystallized into what the American Psychiatric Association (APA) currently calls ADHD. The fact that the symptoms we today call ADHD have had so many different names over the years suggests that it may be reasonable to expect that the language describing these childhood problems may change yet again in the future.

The epidemiological breakdown of ADHD in the United States and Canada is constantly changing, partially due to the fact that ADHD comprises so many symptoms, but also because the presentation of the data of those who are afflicted tends to serve the interests of the researcher. The "anti-Ritalin" camp, for example, has estimated that 10 to 12 percent of school-age children are diagnosed with ADHD and take medications (Breggin 1995; also see Moore 1998), while proponents of Ritalin treatment estimate that only 3 to 5 percent of school-age children are diagnosed with the disorder (Barkley 1995a).

As for gender, the epidemiological breakdown has an estimated male-female ratio of five-to-one (Arnold 1995, 1996), but the prevalence of the disorder in females remains unclear[2] (Biederman et al. 1999). In addition, the difference in rates of ADHD is marked when clinic-referred data are compared with community samples; male-female ratios are ten-to-one and three-to-one, respectively (Gaub and Carlson 1997). As for race, recent studies argue that the cases of ADHD in African American children are proportional to the cases in the white population, though the data from such studies do not make the imperative distinction between clinic-referred and community samples.[3]

These and numerous other examples highlighted in this book show that ADHD is a bone of contention. It should not be regarded as a medical falsehood or, conversely, as a medical reality. This perspective is unsuitable for those determined to debunk medical practitioners or, conversely, those who wish to champion the cause of modern medicine. One of the goals of a genealogical perspective is to step outside of the "either/or" etiological debate and objectify the debate itself or, more specifically, to objectify *parts* of the debate. Instead of proposing an ontology of ADHD, it would be more pertinent to examine the discourse that has constituted ADHD as an object in the same spirit as Michel Foucault's genealogical studies,[4] which "will cultivate the details and accidents that accompany every beginning; it will be scrupulously attentive to their petty malice; it will await their emergence, once unmasked, as the face of the other" (1984, 80). Genealogy does not force continuity among historical events; rather, it sniffs out the dynamics of the "petty malices" that constitute the beginnings of an object of knowledge. From Foucault's perspective, the discussion of any object of knowledge begins by paying attention to the aggressive politics between differing perspectives toward that object.

Foucault's (1965, 1973, 1977) studies of institutions, such as the mental asylum, the hospital, and the prison, provide the starting point for a critique of the knowledge bases and practices of such institutions. Such studies demonstrate that the professional and lay influence of these institutions results from how knowledge systems make their way into institutional practice. This particular assertion shows a tremendous fit with the social dynamics that characterize the informal/formal duality analyzed in the sociology of mental health. As mental disorders, for example, become visible to the medical establishment and therefore legitimate objects of study, they form the power base of institutions. The project of genealogy, then, is to explain how these knowledge systems came to be and to show how they affect perceptions and behavior in the lay world.[5] Given its goals, a genealogical perspective is particularly effective in analyzing mental disorders. Ian Hacking's examination of Multiple Personality Disorder (MPD) in *Rewriting the Soul* (1995) and Allan Young's analysis of Post-Traumatic Stress Disorder (PTSD) in *The Harmony of Illusions* (1995) reflect Foucault's influence but also represent a considerable advancement of genealogical methods, and new directions of study in mental health. In *Harmony* and *Rewriting*, neither author makes an etiological or philosophical commitment to the mental illness in question. Instead, both authors elaborate a narrative of each of these mental illnesses, methodically presenting historical and contemporary discourses that address them. With each text, the reader is left well informed on the etiological, symptomatic, and epidemiological discourses that make up MPD and PTSD. Because neither author takes sides, both are free to address all discussions of MPD and PTSD, rather than ignoring points that may undermine a central argument.

The work of Hacking and Young represents contemporary examples of Foucault's analysis of the shape and dynamics of knowledge systems. In addressing discourse, Foucault studied the ways in which different disciplines or people within the same discipline contest objects of knowledge, and the ways lay people are affected by the institutional and discursive manifestations of those disciplines. This position was a way for Foucault to offer an alternative to the concept of ideology, which was such a deterministic force for his Marxist critics: "I would like to substitute this whole play of dependencies for the uniform, simple notion of assigning a causality; and by suspending the indefinitely extended privilege of the cause, in order to render apparent the polymorphous cluster of correlations" (Foucault in Barrett 1991, 130). Ideology, from a classic Marxist perspective, is dispensed unilaterally from those in positions of economic power to the masses, which internalize these belief systems and act in accordance with them. Sociological examinations of mental health discuss notions of mental disorders as ideological. Corporate and medical realms, it is argued, control public perception; hence, the idea of a mental disorder is dispensed to a susceptible public similarly to the way economic systems dispense beliefs and values.

Genealogical perspectives objectify the process through which statements are made about a mental illness and, to a lesser degree, the methods that propel those statements. Hence, those who provide genealogical accounts of a mental disorder are inclined to discuss the phenomenon at hand as a result of "narratives" crafted by the warring factions in the discursive field.[6] The use of the term "narrative," many argue, reduces a mental illness to a kind of story rather than a lived social reality. At this point, "empirically based" social science tends to withdraw support from genealogical methods because the experience of mental disorder is not articulated in humanistic terms. Genealogical studies become relegated to the amorphous research category of "postmodern methodology" and are argued to be more suitable for literary criticism and cultural studies forums.

Such accounts have a tremendous variability in the types of "data" with which they engage. This stems from the theoretical positions about the discursive field, specifically that this field is enormous—to the point of being impossible to quickly summarize in one study—and is comprised by extreme variability. Genealogists scrutinize the sets of statements to be objectified at the admitted exclusion of others. There is a sort of faith that they will examine the discourses that appear the most dominant in a contemporary understanding of mental disorder (i.e., an examination of neurological discourses in relation to disorders such as ADHD, schizophrenia, and depression) and analyze such a disorder in terms that contemporary social actors can understand. This is an exciting methodological space. Genealogy exemplifies the basic principles of inductive research, defying many of the ideas of research design, hypothesis creation/testing, theory generation, and so on, but frees a researcher to explore data sources that might otherwise be ignored.

Through focusing on a history of multiple discourses, genealogy promotes a "less-taken-for-granted" perspective on mental illness. Issues of validity become secondary to another analytical context in which discourses are placed within a political arena, portrayed as working within and against each other, always in motion, always propagating new sets of statements. Articulating the constant and seemingly arbitrary shifts in discursive motion, genealogy subverts notions of truth or even the notion of "progress" towards some semblance of truth. This has been interpreted as a "political aim" of genealogy, not because it seeks to invalidate a discourse as "self-serving," or "conspiratorial," but because such an analysis demystifies contemporary dominant discourses.

For sociologists who wish to undermine dominant narratives of mental illness, this method is highly disconcerting. Perhaps part of the reason for this is that their own discourses about a mental disorder—for example, ones which invoke a social etiology—may also be objectified by genealogy's methods. Social determinism cannot reign supreme within a genealogical framework. Because genealogy eliminates the efficacy of alternative discourses, it is a methodology subject to considerable criticism. Hence, borrowing from Susan Sontag, Nancy Fraser (1989, 64-65) playfully calls Foucault's genealogy a great "lover" but terrible "husband," and Jürgen Habermas (1984, 253), who redefines genealogy as "genealogical historiography," calls the method "cynical."

I believe this cynicism may be avoided if the discourses of ADHD are grounded in their empirical relationship to everyday experience. The bulk of this book, therefore, is devoted to showing how the experiences people associated with ADHD have are connected to the various and sundry ADHD discourses that are found in the medical and popular literature. The best way to undertake this connection between discourse and experience is through soliciting actual accounts from people associated with ADHD and allowing them to convey their own experiences. At numerous places throughout this book, I draw connections between the experiences that are articulated by such people in the interviews and those discussions that have determined why these experiences are interpreted as they are. For example, in addressing clinicians' uncertainty about the ADHD diagnosis, I draw attention to the ongoing debate between psychodynamic and neurological views toward ADHD symptoms that began in the 1930s; in exploring why teachers have become proficient "suspectors" of ADHD in their classrooms, I focus on some of the education discourse that admonishes teachers to operate in more of a clinical capacity in locating mentally disordered children; in exploring parents' understanding of the "paradoxical effect" of medications, I offer a detailed analysis of that discussion in the medical literature and show how that discussion has made its way into lay understandings.

Interviewing: Respondent Profile and Methods

Parents, teachers, clinicians, and children were recruited for this study over an eighteen-month period beginning in August 2001, from two North American cities with populations of roughly 500,000 and 200,000. As a starting point of this sample, parents were recruited from a variety of locations, including Children and Adults with Attention Deficit Hyperactivity Disorder (CHADD) meetings and support groups for parents of children with learning disabilities. Over the course of this research I attended numerous ADHD-oriented meetings and was even invited to one CHADD group as a guest speaker on sociological understandings of ADHD. In recruiting respondents from meetings that were not open to the public, the facilitators of such meetings were asked to pass out a flyer clarifying the nature of this research—an approach which proved to be effective when potential respondents could not be directly contacted. As this project solicited accounts about children who are already perceived to be vulnerable, it was imperative that appropriate measures be taken to dispel perceptions of this research as a threat (Blum 1952) and of me as an invasive outsider (Becker 1956; Trice 1970). Since such perceptions can gravely affect interview accounts and respondent recruitment, considerable effort was expended to be as open about the nature of this research project as possible. In particular, I wanted respondents to understand that I was neither "judging" their relationship to ADHD nor conducting any type of clinical experiment. Such declarations on my behalf aided in my being perceived as a person "in the know" (Goffman 1959) and greatly helped to elicit the necessary everyday experience (see Fontana and Frey 2000) or "life story" (Cruikshank 1998) of those involved with the social dynamics of ADHD. Further, being more open with the people I wished to interview reduced some of the pitfalls associated with taking an undue amount of "researcher privilege" (Denzin 2000).

Respondent Profile[7]

Ninety people participated in this study, including thirty parents, twenty-five teachers, twenty-six clinicians, and nine ADHD children. Respondents from all groups were recruited according to a "snowball approach" (Biernaki and Waldorf 1981; Marshall 1996), denoting that the sample grew as respondents referred me to others understood to have experience with ADHD.

Representing a plethora of occupations, parent respondents ranged from twenty-seven to fifty-one years of age, and their ADHD-diagnosed children ranged from six to seventeen years of age. Twenty-six of the parent respondents reported having boys with ADHD, and four respondents had girls with the disorder.[8] Twenty-five of the parent respondents stated that their children were taking or had taken some type of stimulant medication. Twenty-one of the parent respondents were female, and nine were male.

Of the nine children I was given parental permission to interview, only seven are presented. Two of the child respondents were simply too young to actively participate in the interviewing process. In such cases, the accounts parents provided suffice to describe these children's circumstances. The excerpts from the seven interviews I have presented here are with older children, many of whom have lived with the ADHD diagnosis for a considerable length of time. The age range of these child respondents was eleven to seventeen years. All seven were either taking or had taken stimulant medications to manage their ADHD. At the time of the interviews, four of the children—three boys, age twelve, fourteen, and seventeen, and one girl, age fourteen—had ceased taking stimulant medications, whereas the other three children—three boys, age ten, eleven, and thirteen—were still taking stimulants.

Teacher respondents ranged in age from twenty-eight to sixty-four years and included fourteen males and eleven females. Representing fourteen different schools, the grades teachers taught ranged from pre-school to tenth grade. Nine of the respondents taught mixed grade levels, primarily because they were the special education teacher at their school and provided special assistance to children from all grade levels.

Clinician respondents, defined in this study as people who are integral in making formal diagnoses and prescribing methods of treatment for ADHD, ranged from thirty-one to sixty years of age. Ten were female and sixteen male. A cross-section of clinical professions are represented here, including clinical psychologists, psychiatrists, pediatricians, general practitioners, family therapists, one psycho educational assessor, and one registered nurse who was a manager of a hospital clinic that exclusively diagnoses and treats ADHD.

Interviewing Procedure

Parents proved to be crucial gatekeepers who invariably held information about clinicians and educators who were close to their ADHD-diagnosed children. Allowing parents to be a referral source helped to avoid the arduous random sampling of clinician and teacher populations. Prior to the interview, parents were asked who their children's teacher(s) and clinician(s) were at the time of their diagnosis or which clinicians and teachers they knew to have significant experience in dealing with ADHD. These potential teacher and clinician respondents were contacted by phone and subsequently mailed an introductory letter summarizing the purposes of the research. After receiving the introductory letter, all adult respondents were required to acknowledge receiving a form guaranteeing that the data obtained in the interview process would be held in strict confidence and that any publication or presentation of the material would protect respondent anonymity.

Completed over the phone or in person, interviews (all of which lasted between twenty and ninety minutes) were initially structured around a schedule designed for each respondent group but were allowed to take on an informal, conversational tone in many cases. In an effort to avoid "waivering calibrations" (Webb at al. 1966, 22), responses were taken down in note form and read back to the respondent in order to ensure that what was meant would be reflected in the documented interview. The interview data were analyzed according to a grounded theory approach (Glaser and Strauss 1967; Glaser 1978; Strauss and Corbin 1997), and when the respondent sample grew to around fifty participants, specific themes began to emerge, revealing a degree of sample saturation in the data set.

Excepting clinicians, most of the people I interviewed do not hold a sophisticated etiological position toward ADHD. Indeed, most had only a basic understanding of ADHD before the disorder became a professional or personal issue for them. Such people are not the ones selling a new book or a new treatment but are instead those who simply want what is best for themselves, their children, students, and patients. As their stories are presented, I will make great effort to demonstrate how their interpretations of ADHD relate to the decades-old discourse of ADHD. Though this book should be regarded as a tapestry that shows the interconnection between ADHD discourse and everyday experience, I do not want to lose sight of the fact that people are not automata, simply following the dictates of medical science, but are agents in the construction of their own experiences. If this book revealed one thing, it would be that people are certainly influenced by the authoritative voices of sociology, psychology, and psychiatry, but more importantly, people provide that authority in the first place.

Content Summary

With the exception of chapter 2, which explores some of the early concepts for ADHD, this book is organized around three themes, each of which is devoted to a particular respondent group. Chapters 3 and 4 are devoted to clinicians; chapters 5 and 6 are devoted to teachers; and chapters 7 and 8 are devoted to parents and children. This book concludes with a brief chapter that elucidates some of the greater theoretical contributions of this study and directions we may take in the future.

As a history of "pre-ADHD" medical concepts, and written largely in response to the paucity of historical information that has been assembled and published on the disorder, chapter 2 elucidates the historical-discursive context for contemporary understandings of ADHD. Focusing on the medical concepts of idiocy, imbecility, and *encephalitis lethargica* in the late nineteenth and early twentieth centuries, this chapter illustrates how morally inept and unruly children became viewed through a medical lens. Of particular concern in this chapter is the work of George F. Still (1902), regarded by most publishing in the field as the first to draw medical attention to ADHD. I argue here that Still's suspicions of morally challenged children having a "morbid condition" were themselves situated within the greater discussions of imbecility during that time. This chapter also claims that the exploration of the psychological aftereffects of *encephalitis lethargica* infections in the 1920s began a particular neurological interest in childhood deviance.

Chapter 3 analyzes how clinicians interpret ADHD causes and how they use the American Psychiatric Association's *Diagnostic and Statistical Manual of Mental Disorders* (*DSM IV*) (1994) in diagnosing the disorder. An in-depth discussion of the many differences between psychodynamic and neurological perspectives will be provided in conjunction with analyses of how clinicians are influenced by these perspectives. This chapter explores the considerable uncertainty regarding whether or not ADHD can actually be located within the brain and the international response to the neurologically dominant perspectives in North American psychiatry. My contention is that much of this uncertainty makes its way into clinical practice and is demonstrated through clinicians' concerns with *DSM IV* and also in the various and contradictory ways clinicians describe the "real" cause of ADHD.

Chapter 4 is an analysis of how clinicians interact with those parties mostly responsible for the suspicion of ADHD (usually teachers) and the parents of ADHD children. The specific ways in which clinicians are approached by school representatives with suspicions of an ADHD student are explored, as are the ways clinicians implement ADHD treatments. As the interviews reveal, many clinicians see themselves as a "means to an end" for teachers, denoting that clinicians' credentials are used to place unruly children on medication, regardless of what the child's *true* problems may be. Indeed, some clinicians express significant conflict with teachers, often contending that teachers overstep their professional boundaries by "practicing medicine" in their classrooms. With regard to the application of treatment techniques, this chapter emphasizes the role stimulant medications play in the treatment of ADHD and analyzes clinicians' approaches to medication within the broader historical discussion of stimulants that began with Charles Bradley in 1937. Although stimulant medications remain the predominant method for treating ADHD, clinicians administer such medications with considerable caution, often expressed as ambivalence toward such treatment measures.

Chapter 5 begins the analysis of teacher interviews by exploring how educators conceptualize ADHD children, detect such children within the classroom, and present assessments to parents. Among the numerous characterizations teachers offer are descriptions of ADHD children as volatile and antagonistic toward teacher and curricular authority. This chapter examines the interest teachers have with ADHD through exploring the literature that advocates strategies for teachers to become better at suspecting the disorder. The manner in which teachers present their suspicions to parents through school-based teams demonstrates the growing clinical role of schools. Elaborating the dichotomy between informal and formal suspicion, the classroom is a realm of semiformal suspicion, where teachers apply clinical knowledge about ADHD in a way that thwarts opinions that they may be inappropriately practicing medicine.

Chapter 6 focuses on the pedagogical responses that teachers employ in dealing with ADHD. Further illustrating how they frame the nature of ADHD children, teachers describe the steps by which they modify assignment structure and the academic and social expectations of ADHD children. As many teachers convey, the following of school protocols in response to ADHD is highly problematic because such procedures largely do not exist or have unclear standards. The lack of uniformity teachers convey regarding school protocols for dealing with ADHD is an extension of the greater diagnostic uncertainty that surrounds the disorder. As many teachers articulate, the pedagogical response to ADHD is implicit in the standards of being a generally effective teacher. This chapter concludes with a discussion of how the pedagogical response to ADHD is a gendered phenomenon, as boys are diagnosed with ADHD much more often than girls. Teachers offer revealing insights regarding ADHD and gender; for example, some convey that the school environment is largely unsympathetic to traditionally "boy behavior" and tends, therefore, to pathologize boys more than girls.

Founded upon a medicalization framework, chapter 7 analyzes how a child's informal troubles become eventually seen as deviance. The first part of the book to explore parents' and children's experiences with ADHD, this chapter draws on a "micro-politics of trouble" perspective to analyze how parties organize themselves around a trouble and cooperatively frame it as medical. Two of the primary troubles parents and children describe are the academic and social struggles that occur within the school context. For some parents, the notion that their children's struggles were part of a "phase" and therefore resolvable through the natural course of events gave way as those problems persisted and increased in intensity. This chapter is a commentary on how parents negotiate between informal and formal modes of suspicion and reveals the tremendous burdens that are placed upon parents as they exercise agency in interpreting why their children have the problems that they do.

Chapter 8 concludes the analysis of interviews by examining how parents, upon finding out their children have ADHD, become informal experts on the disorder and use this expertise in interpreting the meaning of the disorder. Overall, the meaning that is attributed to ADHD is largely a function of parents' perceived uniqueness of their children: parents find many ways to assert that their children are exceptional or resilient, even in the presence of the ADHD diagnosis. Explored at length here are the ways in which suspecting parties first introduce parents to resources containing facts about ADHD. As it is repeatedly discussed by parents as one fact that convinced them that ADHD was real, the discourse of the "paradoxical effect" of stimulant medications is explored in-depth. In addition, some of the prevalent "alternative discourses" are a significant part of materials parents use, including the discussions that connect ADHD to diet and/or television and video games. These are also examined at considerable length.

This book concludes with a discussion of how genealogical and medicalization approaches to the study of mental disorder find valuable points of convergence if applied to qualitative data sources, such as interviews. An analytical point that is important to emphasize is that the way people organize themselves around deviance and, in the case of ADHD, medicalize childhood misbehavior is largely a function of the discourses that have shaped their professional and personal perceptions. The social roles that surround ADHD and prompt the mechanisms of medicalization are rooted in a broader sociohistorical framework, which is partially composed of discourse. Future studies of mental disorder may be well served by this perspective, which could engender a larger historical discussion alongside analyses of empirical data.

Notes

1. Hyperkinesis was the dominant medical term for what is today called a "hyperactive subtype" of ADHD. An extensive breakdown of past and current ADHD nomenclature will be presented at length in subsequent chapters.

2. The gender discrepancy in ADHD cases is a major obstacle to a neurological etiology of this disorder. The fact that so many more boys than girls appear to have the disorder fails to be adequately explained by the neurological discourse, which so readily contends ADHD is physiological. For example, no substantial study brings forth scientific evidence to demonstrate that the gender discrepancy in ADHD cases is related to differences in male and female endocrine systems. Furthermore, sociology and cultural anthropology have established that within the realm of gender we see discernible forms of social constructionism. Indeed, the social dynamics associated with gender are ignored when it comes to clinical discussions of ADHD difference in boys and girls.

3. Reliable data that describe the incidence of ADHD by other racial categories, such as Hispanic, Asian, and Native American, are not available. Class-specific data are also unavailable.

4. See especially *Discipline and Punish* (1977) and *The Birth of the Clinic* (1973) as examples of this method.

5. The relationship between institutionally based knowledge and practices and the everyday world is what Foucault (1978) calls the "extradiscursive dependency."

6. Young, Allan. *The Harmony of Illusions: Inventing Post-Traumatic Stress Disorder*. Princeton, NJ: Princeton University Press, 1995.

7. As this study is based on intensive interviewing and draws from a relatively small sample in comparison to other methodological procedures that are better suited to the development and analysis of data from larger samples, it should be noted that certain social variables would be inadequately addressed if analyzed in this forum. Hence, studies cross-tabulating race, class, and gender and the diagnosis of ADHD may be better suited to a quantitative approach and would indeed be a welcome addition to the sociological study of ADHD. As will be seen in following chapters, excerpts from respondents mention age and occupation. This is not meant to imply an analysis of these variables but rather to simply show more of a human face to the respondent group. This same method of description is also used in the award-winning work of David Karp (1996).

8. The large proportion of male children with ADHD resonates with the clinical literature addressing ADHD and gender. Though the actual ratio of ADHD boys to ADHD girls remains uncertain, it is widely accepted in clinical circles that the vast majority of ADHD children are boys (Arnold 1995, 1996; Biederman et al. 1999).

Chapter Two

Before We Called It ADHD:
Idiocy, Imbecility, and *Encephalitis Lethargica*[1]

ADHD is an acronym embedded in popular culture, yet the history of ADHD is little discussed in popular and academic literature. Brief histories of the disorder have been provided by researchers in the ADHD field (Kessler 1980; Barkley 1990, 1991, 1997) and also by those who are skeptical of the ADHD diagnosis (Schrag and Divoky 1975). Shrag and Divoky, for example, treat the history of ADHD as one of "child control." On the other hand, historical accounts by Kessler and Barkley discuss the history of ADHD as one characterizing the progress of modern clinical practice, slowly honing its nomenclature to greater levels of scientific validity and practical effectiveness. The medical concepts predating ADHD, such histories imply, are stepping stones to increased knowledge and decreased human suffering. In addition to being markedly brief, both of these sorts of historical accounts are plainly ideological and appear only as they benefit author agendas.

The most common starting point for historical accounts of ADHD is a series of lectures given by George Frederic Still in 1902. Both skeptics of ADHD validity (Shrag and Divoky 1975, Breggin 1998) and advocates (Barkley 1990, 1997) trace the lineage of the study of ADHD to these lectures. Though this chapter will address the work of Still, I will not begin a conceptual history of ADHD with his lectures. Instead, I will predate Still's address and discuss the clinical distinction between two nineteenth-century medical terms: *idiocy* and *imbecility*, and focus on how the discussion of *imbecility* marked a point at which nervous disease diagnoses were made in response to individual ineptitude. *Imbecility* became part of the nomenclature enabling medical practitioners to question the mental health of persons who were not drastically maldeveloped or mentally handicapped. Medical discourse also addressed the moral aspects of imbecility, eventually positing the concept of the "moral imbecile" around the beginning of the twentieth century. As will be shown, imbecility was a medical diagnosis that included persons who could not function within conventional institutional structures and engaged in behaviors that were socially inappropriate, often criminal. This included, to a large extent, the behaviors of children—something in which Still took particular interest.

This chapter will examine the work of Still as a conglomeration of the many medical discourses surrounding imbecility and morality in the late nineteenth and early twentieth century. After examining the discourse of imbecility and idiocy, I will demonstrate how Still's work was significant for the medical study of child immorality. It will be argued that Still was the first to link notions of moral imbecility to children, even though he failed to provide an official diagnosis for this childhood behavior.

This history of the early ideas that laid the groundwork for today's understanding of ADHD concludes by exploring the medical establishment's discussion of *encephalitis lethargica* (EL) in children during the 1920s. According to Kessler (1980) and Barkley (1990, 1997), the medical discussion of EL, or "sleepy sickness," is crucial to understanding the formulation of the concept of ADHD. The psychological sequelae of this disease were supposed to be the root of a litany of childhood behavioral problems, including many of the things we today associate with ADHD: inability to concentrate, overactivity, impulsivity, and so on. The nomenclature that addressed the residual effects of EL realized much of Still's earlier suspicions. What Still had suspected as an organic defect or lesion in immoral children was made into a clinical reality by those who studied EL.

Idiocy versus Imbecility

Today the notions of both idiocy and imbecility are so popularized that their clinical meanings have all but been forgotten. Interestingly, those who wrote about idiocy and imbecility in the medical literature of the 1870s also struggled to keep their meanings within the confines of medical nomenclature (see Ireland 1877). The idiot was a type of person who needed to be clarified and understood as a medical phenomenon, not jeered at and mocked as a social misfit. The term was not to be used as a catch-all typology for someone deemed socially inept. The concept of the imbecile largely functioned to clarify the diagnosis of idiocy and later occupied its own place in mental health nosology. William Ireland (1877, 1) provides a distinction between the two terms:

> Idiocy is mental deficiency or extreme stupidity, depending
> upon malnutrition or disease of the nervous centres, occurring
> before birth or before the evolution of the mental faculties in
> childhood.
>   The word imbecility is generally used to denote a less de-
> cided degree of mental incapacity. Thus, when a man distin-
> guishes between an idiot and an imbecile, he means that the
> mental capacity of the former is inferior to that of the latter.

Imbecility here denotes a condition much less severe than that of idiocy,
but the extent of the difference between the two terms is unclear. The
idiot is presented as someone who has an organic disorder of some kind,
the onset of which occurs at the earliest phases of life. The imbecile is
someone with a lesser degree of the same symptoms as the idiot. The
imbecile can certainly demonstrate "mental deficiency" or "stupidity,"
yet not as severely as the idiot.

British physician Charles Mercier (1890) expanded on the distinction
between these two mental aberrations. Lumping both idiocy and imbecility into the category of "congenital mental deficiency" or *dementia naturalis* (286), Mercier provided a more sophisticated analysis of the distinction between the two diagnoses. His analysis rested upon notions of
the successive stages of mental development:

> The first thing the child learns is to avoid physical danger—to
> keep from falling into the water, running against obstacles,
> burning and cutting itself, and all forms of physical injury.
> ...when the activities answering to this class of circumstances
> has been thoroughly acquired, then, and not till then, begins
> the acquisition of those activities by which the livelihood is to
> be earned. Then begins the formal process of education, which
> is the first step in fitting the individual to get his living. When
> this has been done, when sufficient time has been spent daily
> in the acquisition of these activities, then what remains over
> can be devoted to recreation and other purposes (289-90).

Mercier claimed that the development of certain faculties throughout the
early part of life enabled the individual to function at increasingly higher
levels. The lowest level of functioning is denoted by the individual's
ability to display basic self-preservation, thereby avoiding physical injury. The higher levels of functioning that distinguished between normal
and defective persons denoted commitments to institutions deemed cru-

cial to increasing one's quality of life, including receiving an education and finding adequate employment.

Mercier (1890, 290) claimed that the idiot was a type of individual who demonstrated poor development at the most basic level of human existence. Idiots were to be watched and cared for; they were a danger to themselves because of their lack of awareness of their surroundings. Imbeciles represented a slightly higher, though still inadequate, level of development:

> In idiocy the deficiency is still greater. The imbecile fails to adapt himself to his vital environment, he fails to complete the second step in his intellectual development; but he surmounts completely the first step, that which enables him to adapt himself to his *physical* environment [emphasis in original].

Imbeciles could avoid dangerous moving objects but could not be adequately educated to make a living. In this sense, the imbecile personified a failure to meet social and institutional demands.

Imbecility as a category of mental defect became widely known in the medical community as a specific phenomenon not to be confused with the more obvious and impairing condition of idiocy. A medical definition of imbecility was adopted in 1912 by the Royal College of Physicians in England, which claimed that an imbecile "is incapable from mental defect, existing from birth or from an early age, (a) of competing on equal terms with his normal fellows, or (b) of managing himself or his affairs with ordinary prudence" (Goddard 1915, 12).

Moral Imbecility

The ineptitudes described in the discussion of imbecility were eventually linked to an individual's inability to display moral restraint and lawful behavior. In what became known as "moral imbecility"[2] medical practitioners conceptualized the acquisition of morality as a problem of human biological development. William Ireland (1900, 287) provides a description:

> We now and then read of a "moral imbecility," a variety of the unhappy invention styled "moral insanity," originally intended to signify a total want of moral feelings as proved by reckless and shameless conduct without any intellectual impairment.

> . . . The title "moral imbeciles," however, is so far correct that there are certain children who show from the beginning a proneness to evil, a callous selfishness, and a want of sympathy with other people, which is the most striking part of this disorder.

This passage represents much of the literature addressing moral imbecility around the turn of the century and presents a new direction of study for medical science. The inability to demonstrate moral behavior, in that it fell under the rubric of imbecility, could be understood as a medical problem. Ireland (1900, 288) describes a case of moral imbecility—a boy, K.N., housed in a hospital dormitory:

> The first symptom of insanity was his smashing of panes of glass in the passage and other places where he would not be readily noticed. When asked why he did so he said that he liked to see the glass fly. This went on for about six months. One day he took out of his pocket a knife which he had got hold of and deliberately made an incision in a boy's hand.

The imbecile represents one more piece in the historical tapestry of discourse that has objectified the "nature" of the criminal, the uneducated, or the undisciplined. In *Discipline and Punish* (1977) Foucault discusses such processes of objectification as constructing the "modern soul." This modern soul represents the perceived essence of those who engaged in deviant behavior—an essence believed to be understandable and malleable only through the administration of scientific techniques. Foucault's work in *Discipline* is mainly credited with analyzing modern science's examination and objectification of the criminal (whom Foucault calls *homo criminalis*), but this process of seeking the essence of the deviant through scientific study encompasses virtually anyone who has persistent troubles with conventional institutions. Within the discourse of imbecility during the late nineteenth and early twentieth centuries, particular attention is given to children. An examination of medicine's focus upon the moral propensity of children is crucial in establishing a bridge between these early discussions and the gradual unfolding of the discussion of ADHD. Much like *homo criminalis*, ADHD children represent an object of study who could not fit into the institutional frameworks of everyday life and need to be reconstituted and made corrigible in order to meet the demands of these institutions.

Moral imbecility evolved as a concept both medically and legally. It was formally included in the British Mental Deficiency Act of 1913, constituting a class of "Persons who from an early age display some permanent mental defect coupled with strong vicious or criminal propensities on which punishment has had little or no deterrent effect" (Tredgold 1917, 43). The continued failure of reformative intentions of punishment, or the threat thereof, led many medical practitioners to believe that the moral imbecile represented a case of incorrigibility in the face of the disciplinary mechanisms of that time period. Hence, there was an increasing pressure on the medical establishment to conceptualize and reconceptualize moral imbecility in an effort to apply effective treatment techniques.

Part of the later conceptualization of the moral imbecile involved the discussion of this type of imbecile being, in many cases, of normal or even superior intelligence. The moral imbecile, physicians argued, was a more complex creature than physicians had initially thought. Physician Alfred Tredgold (1917, 43), in an article on moral imbecility, states: "Many undoubted moral imbeciles are so cunning, so plausible, and so seemingly intelligent, that mental defect, as normally understood, would appear to be, and in truth, is, quite out of the question." In an article covering the same topic two months later, Charles Mercier (1917, 303) states: "I would go farther than Dr. Tredgold, and say that some moral imbeciles are not only seemingly intelligent, but really intelligent. I have met more than one who have engaged me in a battle of wits, in which I did not win every round." These observations by medical practitioners is ironic given the conceptual history of imbecility. The imbecile was generally defined as someone who functioned at a lower level than his/her peers, perhaps just a step or two above the idiot. The concept of the moral imbecile was able to abandon these "human development" presuppositions because it represented a specific type of ineptitude coexisting with other human faculties—those of intelligence, emotion, and physical skill—that could be regarded as normal.

Examining the Work of George F. Still

George F. Still's work must to be understood within the context of the aforementioned discourse of imbecility and idiocy. His 1902 discussion of moral control in children as a medical problem rode the crest of the discussion of imbecility by his peers and no doubt reflects their influence. Because of this, Still's work should not be regarded as the point of origin of the medical account of ADHD children. It might be better understood as a product of the dominant medical literature of his time. Moreover, ADHD researcher Russell Barkley (1990) presents Still's research into immoral children as more meticulous than it was, making it seem novel, or avante garde. Still's work, I believe, represents a plea to the medical community rather than a breaking medical discovery.[3]

Still's plea begins in a series of lectures given before the Royal College of Physicians of London in March 1902, in which he proposes a new topic of medical examination:

> Mr. President and gentlemen, the particular psychical conditions with which I propose to deal in these lectures are those which are concerned with an abnormal defect of moral control in children. . . For some years past I have been collecting observations with a view to investigating the occurrence of defective moral control as a morbid condition in children, a subject I cannot but think calls urgently for scientific investigation (Still 1902, 1008).

In this address, Still tentatively hypothesizes the relationship between self-control and the biological propensity for understanding the moral demands of one's environment. He states: "Moral control can only exist where there is a cognitive relation to environment" (1008). Individual morality is a developmental phenomenon, Still argues, that stems from organic functions of the brain. He contends that at a certain age there are biological standards for moral conduct, and to have less moral control than others in a particular age category is a basis for suspecting a pathological condition.[4]

Still (1902, 1009) eliminates mental retardation as a variable affecting this immoral condition. His discussion separates "the idiot" from those with more particular moral difficulties:

> The driveling idiot who recognizes no one, does not distinguish his food, and is little more than a mere automaton stands in little or no cognitive relation to his surroundings and *a fortiori* lacks that higher form of reasoning comparison which we call moral consciousness. Here, therefore, the absence of moral control is complete. Such cases are of interest chiefly as exemplifying one cause of failure of development of moral control; they have otherwise little bearing on the question before us and need not detain us further.

The child with inadequate control of his/her moral faculties, it is argued, should not be confused with the intellectually inferior. This line of reasoning resonates very well with the later literature that separates the morally inferior from the intellectually inferior. As Mercier (1917) and Tredgold (1917) would later do, Still pleads to the medical community to not misunderstand immoral children as being less intelligent than children who demonstrated moral prowess. The immorality Still wishes to address is presented as significantly "too advanced" for visibly deranged or mentally incapacitated children. Immorality in the normal child, at least the child who defied categories like "retarded," is argued to be symptomatic of some larger medical issue. For Still, some of these symptoms included "(1) passionateness; (2) spitefulness-cruelty; (3) jealousy; (4) lawlessness; (5) dishonesty; (6) wanton mischieviousness-destructiveness" (1009).[5]

For Still, these immoral behaviors represented a degree of personal agency on behalf of the children who displayed them. These were not children who, due to being too stupid to understand the moral codes of society, acted out against those codes. These children had a clear understanding of the contents of the law and willfully chose to disregard it. Nameless to modern medicine, these children were too intelligent to be categorized under the established nomenclature of idiocy and too young to be understood as "criminal minds." For Still, as with those researchers who would follow in his footsteps, these were the "other children" who required a more specific understanding through medical examination. Still ultimately questioned whether or not these children represented an entirely new form of idiocy of imbecility: "Lastly, the question must be raised whether we can associate defect of moral control with any particular type or types of idiocy or imbecility—a question of considerable importance, for if it were possible to do so we might hope by a study of these types to find some anatomical basis for this abnormality of function" (1012).

Still's lecture was given during a time when there were other discussions about the biological characteristics of immorality, more specifically, criminal behavior. Lombroso's infamous *L'Uomo Delinquente* (1876), though today regarded as scientifically flawed, was an unquestionable influence upon the medical discussions of morality during this time period. By comparing the morphology of criminals (including the size of the jaw bone, amount of brow pronouncement, and arm length) to that of law-abiding persons, Lombroso elucidated a medical typology to discover criminals. Still's discussion, though obviously a product of its time, differs from Lombroso's. Even as Still comments about the physicality of these children in an effort to make a distinction between them and those in the "normal" population, Still's analysis proposes a different focus of the scientific study of unconventional childhood behavior—an uncharted, *neurological* one. There is an implicit assumption in his idea of the cognitive component of morality that the cause of these immoral behaviors lay hidden inside the mind of the child. The cause of this immorality was unknown and hidden. To understand the cognitive origins of moral pathology would imply a more methodical examination. Though he suspected a specific type of imbecility, Still offered no conclusions about the cause of these moral ineptitudes; his tone is one that seems to recognize the long, hard road ahead for modern medicine. As theoretically unsophisticated as it was, Still's work reflected a passion within medicine, beginning a process of inquiry and debate that has yet to be resolved.

Still's work is significant for the examination of the early discourse surrounding ADHD and represents a break from the more general medical discussions of moral ineptitude because he proposed that children become an object of study. Though ADHD is being increasingly diagnosed in adults, it remains a disorder perceived to almost exclusively afflict the young. Up to the point of Still's address, the elaboration of diagnostic categories—especially those like "moral imbecility"—were not understood in a direct relationship to children. Stemming from the discourse of idiocy and imbecility, Still provided some of the groundwork for a category of mental illness that is specific to potentially delinquent youth.

Encephalitis Lethargica as an Explanation of Youth Delinquency

The medical discussion of *encephalitis lethargica* (EL) in the 1920s is considered an early point in the discussion of specific childhood symptoms that would later be attributed to ADHD (Stewart 1970; Kessler 1980; Cantwell 1981; Barkley 1990). Also known as "sleepy sickness," EL reached epidemic proportions toward the close of World War I. It was a disease unknown to medicine at its outbreak but quickly became a centerpiece of medical attention. Isador Abrahamson (1920a, 17) provides a concise history of the spread of the illness:

News of this strange plague had scarcely escaped from the be-
leaguered Central Empires when the disease itself suddenly
appeared in the outer world. An epidemic which was described by J. H. Mathewson and Oliver Latham, began in February, 1917, in the province of New South Wales, Australia;
whence it spread to Queensland and to Victoria. It persisted
till the following May. . . . On February 11, 1918, the first recognized case occurred in England, and an outbreak followed
which, with remissions, lasted until January, 1919. Then the
disease appeared in Ireland. In 1918 the epidemic was reported as raging also in Uruguay and in Algeria, in Germany
and in Greece. . . .

So far as is known the first recognized case of this epidemic
disease in America entered Mount Sinai Hospital, New York
City, in September 1918.

EL was an often fatal illness characterized by tremendous sluggishness,
hallucinations, and fever, often bringing with it periods of remission—
something doctors viewed optimistically. These remissions were commonly short-lived, and a full relapse of the illness was a common occurrence: "The early optimism I enjoyed quickly perished, and I learned to
dread this disease, so often fatal, not infrequently inflicting permanent
damage on those who survived it, and sometimes bringing in its train
progressive functional deterioration" (Abrahamson 1920b, 428).

What became as significant as the symptoms of the disease itself were
the residual effects of encephalitis (this is what Stryker [1925] calls the
"behavior residuals" of encephalitis; also see Paterson and Spence [1921]
and Hohman [1922]). It was a disease thought to irreversibly damage
many who suffered it, leaving people with extensive physical and mental
impairments. These physical and psychological sequelae came in so
many forms that it was common for neurologists to refer to them as a
syndrome.

EL had as many as twenty-seven different symptoms, including:
"sleep reversals, emotional instability, irritability, obstinacy, lying, thiev-
ing, impaired memory and attention, personal untidiness, tics, depression, poor motor control, and general hyperactivity" (Kessler 1980, 18).
Hardly an elegant diagnosis, EL is significant because it marks a point
where moral and scholastic difficulties are understood through somatic
disease categories. The discussion of EL made a strong break from that
of idiocy and imbecility because it replaced moralistic reasoning with
inquiries that were firmly grounded in physiology.

Franklin G. Ebaugh (1923, 90) describes the sequelae of encephalitis as behavior patterns contrasting with those prior to the encephalitis affliction, ranging from alterations in sleeping and eating patterns to marked oppositional behavior:

> Normal children who were well adjusted in school and home changed abruptly to a state of hyperkinesis, characterized by transient periods of talkativeness, tension states and emotional outbreaks often leading to general incorrigibility and inability to remain in school. . . . One of the patients, a girl aged 10, was difficult to manage. She was noisy, abusive to other children and capriciously depressed. She was "bossy," quick tempered, and impulsive and showed little respect for authority.
> . . . She gave evidence of definite sexual precocity. One boy had streaks of cruelty, and on one occasion stabbed a schoolmate with a knife. Another boy, who formerly had been quiet and orderly, became obscene and masturbated in public.

To Ebaugh, these and other sequelae represented a "total change in the...character and disposition" (Ebaugh 1923, 90) of children who were at one time happily involved in school, family life, friendships, and so on. After the onslaught of the formidable illness, these children exhibited behaviors that not only fell outside the parameters of appropriate behavior within these contexts but also, at times, went directly against them. These sequelae comprised a drastic alteration in personality, commonly represented by actions against accepted institutions, for example, schools: "In three of our patients marked hysterical phenomena were observed. One child developed spells of the functional variety, usually to escape from a difficult situation. The spells consisted of prolonged periods of rapid respirations, the child thus feigning illness in order to stay out of school" (91).

In a later discussion of the sequelae of encephalitis, Roger Kennedy (1924) formulated similar descriptions, citing numerous case studies, each organized according to a particular category of sequelae. Discussing the sequelae described as "Change in Personality and Behavior" (Kennedy 1924, 169), he comments on the state of a 10-year-old:

> a boy aged 10 years was brought to the clinic May 9, 1922, because of nervousness. In March, 1920, he had influenza followed by an acute attack of encephalitis which lasted eight days. . . . He improved gradually and returned to school, but

had to be taken out because he asked so many questions and removed books from other desks to his own.

In September, 1920, another attempt was made to have him attend school, but this was soon given up as he started to steal at random. He took a diamond ring belonging to his sister and disposed of it for an automobile ride (170).

Kennedy's is one of the first accounts that attempts to create a case for these sequelae, especially those concerning defiant behavior, to be understood as a syndrome. He argued that delinquency and other symptoms of post-encephalitic infections in children represented a physiological mechanism. This position remains the dominant perspective of today's neurologically oriented ADHD researchers: ADHD is a syndrome comprising a variety of behaviors with a basic neurological cause. Kennedy states: "This case illustrates the main features to be considered in dealing with children who are suffering from this syndrome. In the first place the absolutely different personality which they display is well exemplified. They are apparently acting in response to a most urgent stimulus, which they are powerless to resist" (Kennedy 1924, 170). Here is the beginning of the discussion of post-encephalitic children as not being responsible for their actions. These children, the medical literature demonstrates, merely act according to an unknown (yet hotly pursued) neurological principle.

Similar to Still's initial discussion of child immorality as a medical problem, Kennedy (1924, 171) also wished to exclude those who are retarded or have some kind of obvious mental defect:

> Second, and perhaps of most importance, is the consideration of mental status. As has been indicated, there is no evidence to show that a considerable proportion of such patients are mentally retarded or deficient. . . .They are moral rather than mental imbeciles. Some of them appear dull and drowsy, but in their antics and behavior they display a cunning that is not commensurate with greatly impaired mental faculties.

The idea that a child could be "dull and drowsy" speaks not to an issue of intelligence but to the dominant understanding of EL. This disease was thought to be characterized by an untimely sluggishness in children that apparently disappeared when they responded to a neurological stimulus. This is a different kind of mental impairment, distinct from retardation, in which afflicted children were described as cunning and calculating.

This is little different from the description of the moral imbecile whom Mercier and others in the late nineteenth and early twentieth centuries considered to be both defective and at the same time have moderate, if not high, intelligence.

Kennedy's perspective, depicting the immoral behavior of the post-encephalitic child as the result of neurological processes, is elaborated by Edward Strecker (1929, 137-8) who made distinctions between two types of behavior exhibited by the post-encephalitic child: (1) "motor" behaviors that were unintentional and outside the control of the child; and (2) "studied" types of conduct that demonstrated conscious effort on the child's part. The author presents examples of each:

> An example of some misconduct of the motor type is as follows: A boy, aged 10, who had acute encephalitis at the age of 7, is described as being overactive, constantly in motion, roaming about the streets at night, wandering about the house at night, whistling and singing; once he dashed up to an infant sister's crib and swung the baby about by the heels. . . In the severe studied type one witnesses such deviations as stealing, forgery, deliberate lying to gain an end, moral lapses and running away, carefully planned and with a definite objective.

Strecker painted two very distinct pictures of this type of post-encephalitic children. On one hand, such children were clearly driven by impulses that fell outside of conscious thought or reason. They slept poorly and were markedly overactive. On the other hand, these children demonstrated certain malice in the things they did. They stole and committed forgery, all with the intent of personal gain. They demonstrated a baffling degree of self-centeredness.

The medical discussion of moral imbecile children portrayed in the late nineteenth century was eclipsed by the much more elaborate discussion of post-encephalitic children. In applying the diagnosis of EL to immoral children, a physiological explanation was provided for immoral, anti-institutional behavior. The discourse on EL is spuriously documented by Kessler, Barkley, Stewart, and others as a place in the history of the gradual sophistication of medical practice, ultimately leading to the "teasing out" of the more correct diagnosis of ADHD. Barkley, for example, claims that children with ADHD in the 1920s were mixed in with the population of those suffering from encephalitic trauma. Due to the rudimentary knowledge of neurology during that time period, EL, Barkley argues, served as a catch-all diagnosis. Such researchers look endearingly at their own discipline's history and claim that medicine had to start somewhere and is gradually becoming more sophisticated, more "correct."

The discussion of EL is significant, not because it drew suspicion to the causal connection between behavior and neurological impulse, but because it problematized myriad symptoms—many of which seemed unrelated—and unified them under a single disease name. Many of these symptoms (impulsivity, concentration difficulties, hyperactivity, and so on) were claimed by neurologists and placed under the rubric of ADHD. From the point in mental health history where EL took center stage as a cause of childhood immorality, up to the current era of ADHD, child psychiatry rested upon a belief that persistently defiant childhood behaviors represented physiological pathology. The specifics of this pathology, including the causes and cures for it, remain a bone of contention both inside and outside of psychiatry.

Notes

1. A different version of this chapter has been previously published as: "The Conceptual History of Attention Deficit Hyperactivity Disorder: Idiocy, Imbecility, Encephalitis and the Child Deviant, 1877-1929." *Deviant Behavior* 22, (2001): 93-115.

2. Charles Mercier (1917) has stated that it was he who coined the term "moral imbecility." The date of the inception of the term could not be found in my research. Due to no findings of another to claim the origin of the term, perhaps credit for placing "moral imbecility" into medical discourse should be awarded at this time to the late doctor.

3. Part of this misrepresentation by Barkley I believe distorts the experimental and conceptual history which has given us the legacy of ADHD. During the time period of Still's writing, there was no large-scale study performed to ascertain the nature of this "ailment." Most of Still's limited number of subjects were part of an institutionalized population subjected to countless socially influenced variables.

4. A standard of self-control as set by a particular age category is still a consistent diagnostic tool in the assessment of ADHD as well as other childhood mental disorders (see American Psychiatric Association 1994, 82).

5. In his discussion of Still's work, Russell Barkley (1990, 4) makes the comment that "Most of these children were impaired in attention and were quite overactive." This is not documented in Still's address.

Chapter Three

Psychodynamic versus Neurological ADHD Narratives: Clinicians Discuss *DSM IV* and the Essences of ADHD

The clinicians I interviewed for this project convey a wide interpretation of the so-called hyperactive and inattentive behaviors that are exhibited by "problem" children. To summarize their approach to ADHD-like behavior, clinicians appear to sympathize with either a psychodynamic or neurological perspective towards the disorder. In adopting a psychodynamic approach, clinicians tend to view ADHD-like symptoms in connection with difficulties between children and their parents, school, church, and so on. ADHD symptoms, from this stance, are children's "behavioral reactions" toward their social environment. Clinicians employing a neurological approach commonly refer to ADHD as a specific brain abnormality. From this perspective, ADHD is regarded in the same manner as any other somatic illness.

The subscription to either a psychodynamic or neurological perspective towards ADHD falls, to some extent, along professional lines. Excepting one highly skeptical pediatrician, most of the testimonials from pediatricians and general practitioners tend to follow a neurological approach to ADHD. Such practitioners evaluate the presence of ADHD in a regimented amount of time and largely believe in the diagnostic efficacy of the American Psychiatric Association's (1994) *DSM IV* criteria for the disorder. Clinical psychologists, psychiatrists, and family therapists, on the other hand, address ADHD in a more nuanced fashion. In adopting a psychodynamic perspective towards ADHD, such clinicians advocate a greater assessment of a child's social circumstances and take considerably longer time in diagnosing the disorder. In accordance with the belief that ADHD is strongly associated with environment, psychodynamically oriented clinicians express a significant amount of skepticism about the use-value of *DSM IV* criteria.

To illustrate the influence of psychodynamic and neurological perspectives in clinical practice towards ADHD, this chapter devotes significant space to a discussion of these perspectives as they have been established in medical and popular literature. Reiterating the genealogical commitment I presented in the introduction, a considerable portion of the history of these perspectives is integral to understanding how current ADHD clinical settings produce, and are produced by, the many discussions that have sought ADHD as their object.

Psychodynamic Approaches to ADHD

Psychodynamic schools of thinking understand ADHD-like childhood behaviors as reactions to environmental conditions rather than as specifically linked to organic causes. This is not to say that all psychodynamic perspectives deny that immoral or disturbing child behavior is caused by organic brain trauma; many publishing in this area certainly present a case for organic brain damage. However, the psychodynamic etiological emphasis is on the degree to which children demonstrate a healthy psychosocial reciprocity with their environment rather than on neurological dysfunction.

Historical Foundations: Anna Freud and Melanie Klein

Two of the most significant figures in the psychodynamic discussion of children are Anna Freud and Melanie Klein. Both Freud and Klein argued that the child mind was developed enough, even in infancy (both believed in the notion of "infant neuroses") to demonstrate marked mental impairment. As psychoanalysts both argued that the key to curing childhood neurosis rested primarily in an understanding of the "latency period" of mental development. Starting around the age of five up to the beginnings of puberty, the highly sexual latency period was believed to be a crucial component in childhood restlessness, mischief, and social detachment. The psyche's adjustment to the latency period manifested itself through various forms of anxiety. For both Freud and Klein, the troublesome period of latency engendered psychic struggle, which commonly appeared as neuroses. Many of the childhood behaviors that are today attributed to symptoms of ADHD psychoanalysts felt were due to an abnormal amount of latency-related anxiety. In Klein's (1932, 144) words:

> Children often show a kind of over-liveliness which often goes along with an overbearing and defiant manner and which people frequently mistake either for a sign of temperament or for disobedience, according to their point of view. Such behavior is, like aggression, an over-compensation for anxiety and this method of modifying anxiety greatly influences the child's character-formation and its later attitude to society. The fidgetiness which often accompanies this over-animation is, in my judgment, an important symptom. The motor discharges which the little child achieves through fidgeting often become condensed at the beginning of the latency period into definite stereotyped movements which are usually lost to view in the general picture of excessive mobility which the child presents.

Behavioral symptoms are secondary to emotional states, Klein argues, that are natural to a phase of child development. "Fidgetiness," in this instance, is a physical overcompensation for the emotional state of anxiety that represents the psychosexual processes of latency. Depending on the other actors involved with the latency period (primarily the child's parents), the severity of the symptoms would vary. A warning is implicit in this passage: the child's overcompensation will solidify itself into a form of "character" or an "attitude to society" in which the world will be treated as antagonistic and dangerous.[1]

Compulsion Neuroses

The "compulsion neurosis" refers to a mental maladjustment in which children and adults feel compelled to repeatedly perform or refrain from particular actions. In the translator's note to Anna Freud's *The Psychoanalytic Treatment of Children* (1946, vi), Nancy Proctor-Gregg defines compulsion neurosis as a condition in which people "cannot (or must) step on the cracks in the pavement." Freud (1926, 6) describes this condition in a six-year-old girl:

> I had to determine whether the difficult, silent and unpleasing nature of the child was due to a defective disposition and unsatisfactory intellectual development, or whether we had here a case of an especially inhibited and dreamy child. Closer observation revealed the presence of a compulsion neurosis, unusually severe . . . together with acute intelligence and keen logical powers.

Described here is a case of what many clinicians today would call an "inattentive ADHD subtype" (APA 1994, 80)[2]. This particular little girl was extremely inhibited in her reactions to others, totally withdrawn and "dreamy." Framed by Freud as having the mental faculties of logic and reason intact, she is also described as being driven by something outside of her will: a *force* of introversion neither the little girl nor Freud can explain. The girl herself has an awareness of this, telling Freud, "I have a devil in me. Can it be taken out?" (Freud 1926, 7).

Later psychodynamic discourse concerning the mental adjustment of children shows minor shifts in nomenclature, though retaining much of the same premises for interpreting neuroses. For example, in a paper presented at the International Institute of Child Psychiatry in Toronto, in August 1954, Beata Rank describes a condition dubbed "atypical development" in preschool children. These are children of normal intelligence who exhibit inappropriate, antisocial behavior. For Rank: "'Atypical development' included impassivity or violent outbursts of anxiety and rage, identification with inanimate objects or animals, and excessively inhibited or excessively uninhibited expression of impulses" (Rank 1954, 491-2). These symptoms represent the psychodynamics of a "fragmented ego"—a refinement of a prior psychoanalytic term, "defective ego," of which Rank is highly critical. Fragmentation denotes an unpredictable relationship between the ego and the world. The relief of antagonism between the individual psyche and the outside world through normal processes of cathexis is not consistently achieved with the fragmented ego. The world becomes a precarious place for this type of ego, which may be prone to violence, utter complacency, or both.

The fragmented ego is argued not to be caused congenitally but through the interactive dynamics of the family system and its effect upon the development of an infant (Rank 1954, 494). Rank argues that these symptoms come from an "infant's unsuccessful struggle to obtain vital satisfaction from his parents" (495) and may cause an increasing psychic isolation of the child from his/her greater social world. Such isolation apparently impedes the development of a normal ego, forcing the child to "pursue only those self-circumscribed activities that provide him with narcissistic and autoerotic gratification without intrusion or interruption from the outside" (495). The manifestations of the fragmented ego represent an extreme form of self-centeredness, requiring the technical intervention of psychotherapy. Furthermore, the "atypical" child is not an isolated system unto him/herself, but part of a poorly functioning family system. Within contemporary psychodynamic understandings of ADHD, it is commonly recommended that the entire family unit undergo psychotherapy.

Less strictly psychoanalytic discussions of childhood mental problems also implicated anxiety as a causal factor in childhood misbehavior but described such anxiety as a result of bona fide brain damage. Renowned for discussing the connection between childhood anxiety and organic brain trauma, Phyllis Greenacre's (1941) work exemplifies the psychological perspective on ADHD children. Citing Greenacre, Lauretta Bender, in "Problems of Children with Organic Brain Disease" (1949), states that behavioral problems of children are a mechanism used to mask a hard-wired, organic difficulty: "The question of anxiety in the brain-damaged child has been very much misunderstood except for the work of Greenacre. The anxiety is of a diffuse type, and the child, too, becomes inured to it and conceals it as he has learned to conceal many of his neurological signs" (Bender 1949, 412). For Bender and Greenacre alike, behavioral problems of organically damaged children are the residuals of a physiological problem—a discussion very similar to that of the psychiatric sequelae of *encephalitis lethargica* addressed in chapter 2. Behavioral outbursts from these types of children are only an effort to mask the anxiety from a failure to fit into the social world as normal children do. This discussion invokes the idea that these children suffer from an organic condition, but denies that this condition is the primary cause of a child's behavioral problems.

Psychodynamic accounts of ADHD-like symptoms argue that the antisocial behavior some children exhibit is a survival mechanism. Over a considerable time after trauma, either through developmental struggle (i.e., latency) or brain injury, these behaviors become crystallized into habits of conduct. The belief is that these habits mask the actual causes of the behavior and hide themselves from the child's own awareness. Due to the fact that ADHD is visible through "habits" rather than a discernible brain lesion, for many clinicians the essence of ADHD remains mysterious.

Today's advocates of the psychodynamic approach stay true to this perspective. Lawrence Diller's *Running on Ritalin* (1998) provides a contemporary example. Often critical of an exclusively neurological perspective on ADHD, Diller presents the case for both the biological and the social factors contributing to the disorder (for a similar yet less critical perspective on ADHD, see Thomas Armstrong, *The Myth of the ADD Child* [1995]). ADHD, although diagnosed carelessly and too often in

Diller's opinion, is presented as an organic reality whose symptoms are merely individual responses to the inadequacies these organic problems foster. In treating ADHD, Diller advocates a philosophy of pediatrics favoring a "family orientation" (Diller 1998, 5) in which it is believed that ADHD symptoms are partially rooted in the social dynamics of the family.

Diller claims that the more difficult cases of ADHD children would be unresponsive to psychotherapy without some form of chemical therapy: "Many of these kids were quite out of control, and intervention with medication (usually Ritalin) was often needed to give other treatments a chance to work" (Diller 1998, 6). This statement contends that the biology of ADHD, if not quelled, is formidable enough to render psychotherapy fruitless. Medications such as Ritalin provide a necessary chemical treatment in which the child can become physically "settled down" enough to be able to undergo psychotherapy. During the therapy process, medicated children can express anxiety about school, family, and friends, hopefully ceasing problem behaviors in these contexts. Chemical therapy alone, Diller warns, will have no staying power if it is not supplemented with some psychotherapeutic approach. He remains highly critical of perspectives on ADHD that have reduced its treatment to the mere "popping of a pill." Diller's position begs the clinical community to add a social sensitivity to its diagnosis and treatment of ADHD.

"I Don't Know What Causes It, but . . ."

It is clear from the sample of clinicians I interviewed that psychodynamic discourse can be highly influential in their practices. Such clinicians claim not to have a definitive knowledge of what causes ADHD. As one clinician says, "I haven't really gone into it," and another, "I am not too sure what current causes are being considered." Underlying this is the belief that if ADHD behaviors cease or are adequately contained, a greater understanding of the physiology of ADHD—if there even is such a physiology—is unnecessary. In addition, clinicians also express that they believe ADHD is not concretely understood at this point by medical science: "I don't really think anyone knows what ADHD is at this point. The research doesn't seem very conclusive, but it's getting better" (clinical psychologist, age forty-two). ADHD is perceived by some to be a disease "in progress," with no solid cause determined at this point. For these clinicians ADHD is still addressed as an actual entity—a *thing* that can be treated. When a theory about the disease process of ADHD is perceived to be inadequate, psychodynamically oriented clinicians choose to emphasize behavior, rather than a disease model, in making ADHD assessments. This focus on behavior, rather than on physiology, exemplifies the treatment of other mental illnesses. As Thomas Szasz (1974) argues, mental illnesses are often "declared" to be what they are, rather than being confirmed through physical evidence.

Despite the APA's attempt to collapse the myriad of childhood behavioral problems into the clinical entity of ADHD, the disorder is still characterized by a wide range of behavioral problems. This litany of problem behaviors has one of two possible effects in the clinic: (1) it may prompt the clinician to easily "see ADHD" in a lot of possible behavioral problems, and hence, make diagnosis easier; or (2) it will make some clinicians cautious as to what constitutes ADHD and what does not. Focusing on the latter instance, many clinicians—especially those practicing in the areas of clinical psychology, psychiatry, or family therapy—felt compelled to take a longer time assessing a child's problems. As one clinical psychologist explained to me: "I am hesitant to provide diagnoses, so I may say 'probable ADHD' until I get more information." From this perspective, rendering a diagnosis of ADHD is expressed as a complicated process requiring considerable information, including testimonials from parents and teachers, extensive records from the child's school, previous clinical assessments, and so on.

Clinicians adopting a multifaceted approach to ADHD state that a certain degree of care must be taken in assessing ADHD so that environmental problems can be separated from organic, brain problems. That is, many clinicians state that it is important to understand the difference between malfunctions that are "hard-wired" into a child's brain and those that are linked to the social environment. The distinction between environmental and organic problems is summarized by one clinician as "primary" and "secondary" diagnoses: "It depends on the circumstances of that child, but they all will get an in-depth clinical interview. I'll try to find out if ADHD is a primary or secondary diagnosis. If it's secondary we probably don't have real ADHD—there's something else going on that needs to be addressed" (clinical psychologist, age fifty-one). Separating a real case of ADHD from psychological problems that only "mimic" the disorder is clearly done in a cautious manner: failure to identify the causes of "secondary diagnoses" raises the risk of misdiagnosis. The perceived separation between real and false ADHD and the methods used to determine this authenticity demonstrate a belief in the neurology of ADHD but validates behavioral problems as legitimate points of concern. In such instances, the methods for treating such problems generally shy away from pharmacology.

The distinction between real ADHD and psychological troubles that mimic the disorder is further articulated by a clinical psychologist whose background is in child neuropsychology. In terms that reflect the continuing debate between psychodynamic and neurological discussions of ADHD, he states: "I typically do a full workup, which includes diagnostic testing, but I also do a full neuropsych battery of tests . . . just to see how the kid operates. During this time I am looking to see if I can separate the neurological stuff from the psychological" (clinical psychologist, age forty-five). In finding out "how the kid operates," this clinician lays claim to having a deeper understanding of the mechanics of a child's thought process. As another clinician states, the knowledge of these mechanics may be crucial to teasing out psychological elements from the diagnostic process: "Before you can really make an assessment, you need to get a feel for how your patients function. That simply takes longer than some people will allow, but you have to see what is a response to a trauma versus what is clearly something real" (psychiatrist, age forty-eight). Clinicians argue that both the organic condition of the brain and the broader social environment of the child can appear behaviorally very similar, yet declarations are ultimately made that separate one from the other. In providing an all-encompassing description for ADHD children, clinicians may argue that it is essential that a specific neurological component be isolated in the diagnosis of the disorder, rendering the child's behavior "out of his/her control."

"I Don't Diagnose. I Just Collect Information"

Clinicians who adopt a psychodynamic position towards ADHD also downplay their roles as those who provide a diagnosis of ADHD and emphasize the development of management programs for specific problems a child may have. These are clinicians who participate in the process of labeling children "ADHD" but do not consider the actual diagnosis to be important. Emphasizing the examination of behaviors only, they instead see themselves as integral to the process of documenting family dynamics and a child's developmental history:

I don't really see children for diagnostic processes. I mean my goal is not to do a diagnosis; that is usually done by a psychiatrist or pediatrician. I do an in-depth family and developmental history, trying to document problems the child may have had in the past. People usually come to me for a more thorough assessment of the child. We really look at the behavior and try to deal with only those behaviors (clinical psychologist, age forty-seven).

As this excerpt demonstrates, an emphasis on behavior can be understood to be more significant than an emphasis on the isolation of a neurological malfunction. Reflecting the rift between psychodynamic and neurological perspectives on the disorder, this clinician implies that the label of ADHD is not nearly as significant as the behaviors that a child exhibits. Hence, she discusses the necessity for "a more thorough assessment of the child" than a one-hour clinical interview can produce. Clearly sympathetic to a psychodynamic rather than neurological interpretation of ADHD symptoms, this excerpt demonstrates a holistic approach to a child's behavioral problems. In this sense, the acquisition of the clinical, neurological label of ADHD is regarded as irrelevant if that label fails to take into account the child's broader social and psychological circumstances.

Another practitioner, a physician emphasizing the synthesis of naturopathic and conventional medicines, provides a similar emphasis on behavior to the exclusion of a neurological label: "I don't really diagnose ADHD. I look specifically at what the child needs. You can label it whatever you want to, but the child needs *something*" (general practitioner, age sixty). The clinical emphasis here is on the immediate needs of the child rather than on the pharmacological treatments mandated by a diagnostic label.

It is arguable that a psychodynamic stance may free a clinician to explore different treatment options for an ADHD-suspected child. There are at least two reasons for this: (1) the child's individual behaviors will be taken into account, including the unique circumstance of his/her family situation, thereby prompting customized forms of treatment; (2) the denial of the over-arching legitimacy of the neurological label of ADHD has potential to focus the treatment effort away from methods (i.e., the administration of stimulant medications such as Ritalin) most strongly associated with the label. There is also, I believe, an identity politics associated with clinicians, separating themselves from the diagnostic process and consequently the label of ADHD. To deny one's role as a "diagnostician" enables a different way of defining oneself in clinical practice. One becomes a professional especially suited to the needs of a child rather than one fitting the child into a preordained conglomeration of symptoms.

Separating oneself from the status of "diagnostician" may be seen as a significant rhetorical strategy, but distancing oneself from the conventional and neurologically influenced methods of diagnosis does not imply a separation from pathologizing childhood behavior. Through the process of what numerous clinicians I interviewed call a "thorough behavioral assessment," including profiling the child's behavior, school records, and teacher accounts, clinicians who do not necessarily believe in ADHD still formally declare that the child is abnormal. Clinicians who do not diagnose yet aggressively pursue avenues of treatment for problem behaviors contribute very much to the labeling process, regardless of the nomenclature they use. This is one nexus point between psychodynamic and neurological perspectives on ADHD: regardless of cause, hyperkinetic and/or inattentive problems are perceived to reflect some degree of abnormality.

Clinician Skepticism toward *DSM IV*

The American Psychiatric Association's (1994) *Diagnostic and Statistical Manual,* fourth edition (*DSM IV*) is the primary text that describes ADHD, and it stems from the neurological work done in the ADHD field. With regard to mental disorders, *DSM IV* represents the neurological establishment, which views the ongoing research into mental disorder as a journey into physiology first and social circumstances a distant second. Therefore, it may be surmised that the extent to which *DSM IV* was reportedly used by clinician respondents partially represents the degree to which neurological maxims were followed. All of the clinicians I interviewed had heard of *DSM IV*, and most of them had great familiarity with the manual.

Psychodynamically inclined clinicians report that they actively use *DSM IV* but argue that it is inadequate in describing ADHD concisely and exclusively. Many of these clinicians describe *DSM IV* as a general guide to ADHD behaviors, but not as the final authority on the subject. When asked if she used *DSM IV* in a suspected case of ADHD, one clinician responds: "Most definitely, when I do make a diagnosis. . . . The *DSM* is a guide; it doesn't account for all of the other variables that go into a diagnosis" (clinical psychologist, age fifty-six). *DSM IV*, it is repeatedly argued in such discussions, is not enough to account for the multiplicity of factors that go into a case of ADHD. More specifically, *DSM IV* may be so general that it fails to acknowledge that ADHD-like behaviors can arise from sources other than bona fide neurological impairment. Another clinician also expresses concern with *DSM IV*, specifically the label of ADHD: "Oh yeah, without a doubt we use it, but we try to look for a lot more than just a diagnostic label. I mean we look at each case really individually because there may be a lot more going on than what the *DSM* can explain" (registered nurse, manager of an ADHD clinic, age thirty-five).

Such sentiments about *DSM IV* also include the perceived financial necessity of the manual. As one clinician comments, *DSM IV* criteria are the basis for third-party recompense: "Insurance companies like to get some kind of diagnosis, and the plain fact is that they do cover ADHD, or just about anything in it [referring to the contents of *DSM IV*]. I guess you might say there is a pressure to use the letters 'A-D-H-D' so that we can move ahead and get a kid treated" (psychiatrist, age forty-eight). More important than the ADHD moniker in such cases is the perceived necessity of treating any child with marked behavioral problems. The belief in the necessity of treatment represents an ethic within the mental health profession. In this sense, *DSM IV* signifies a means to achieving professional obligations.

According to Kirk and Kutchins (1992), the increasing financial pressure that is placed upon mental health practitioners may contribute to "deliberate overdiagnoses" (Kirk and Kutchins 1992, 240), and of course misdiagnoses, of mental disorder. As Kirk and Kutchins (1992) argue, in the event that misdiagnosis occurs, "clients may have good reasons to believe that misdiagnoses are in their best interest" (Kirk and Kutchins, 1992, 240) because a mode of treatment will be financially accommodated. Though they are not articulated in the interviews as "misdiagnoses," there clearly are cases in which the label of ADHD is given for the sole purpose of realizing professional aims that could not be accomplished without the legitimacy of *DSM IV* and the financial compensation that that legitimacy facilitates.

Clinicians also express concerns about some of the specific language that *DSM IV* uses to describe ADHD. This is a more specific criticism of the manual, focusing on the words of *DSM IV* and how they do not always translate into a unified interpretation of behavior. This is especially relevant to whether or not that behavior is perceived as abnormal. As one clinical psychologist explains, "I also think that ADHD is a loaded word. If a kid is unable to stay focused and on task, maybe there are some other reasons for this." ADHD, this clinician contends, may not always be the correct term to apply to problem behaviors, especially those that occur in a scholastic context. She continues to claim that "a lot of times we might need to be focusing on the kid's learning process rather than the problems he may have with attention or concentration," denoting that what *DSM IV* calls ADHD may just be a way of problematizing a different learning style. Addressing the large scope of ADHD symptoms, another clinician states, "I really think that ADHD is a garbage can diagnosis. I wouldn't be surprised if we see the diagnosis get changed within the next couple of years" (family therapist, age fifty-two).

Clinicians also state that they do not use *DSM IV* in cases of suspected ADHD because the language of the manual is not relevant to their clinical perspective on the disorder. For one clinician, the *DSM IV* lacks relevance because the emphasis in his treatment of children is on the collective types of behavior rather than a specific diagnosis:

> I don't [use *DSM IV*] because it's not really relevant to me. When people are referred to me or hear about me through word of mouth, their kids are usually already diagnosed. Again, I just want to look at what the needs of that child are. And, it may very well be Ritalin, but I try to examine some other lines of treatment (general practitioner, age sixty).

The above passage does not denote a complete rejection of the conventional methods for treating ADHD—Ritalin, for example, is not ruled out as an option—yet this clinician uses a certain degree of freedom in interpreting the child's behavior. Similar to clinicians who do not cast themselves as diagnosticians, this clinician exercises the choice to use Ritalin if necessary or explore other options to meet "the needs of that child."

One pediatrician who is entirely skeptical of the ADHD diagnosis finds *DSM IV* irrelevant, because it fails to describe a condition that is visible in contexts outside of school:

> I look at the child's environment, the child's basic needs. If you think about what these needs are, they revolve around home and school because that is where they spend most of their time. These are the areas that need to be evaluated, not the child. ADHD is just plain BS. When a person has diabetes, they have it everywhere they go. With ADHD, we are sup-

posed to believe that these symptoms only exist when they are in school? Nonsense (pediatrician, age forty-nine).

Such skepticism stems from the very specific environments where we suspect that a child may have ADHD. If ADHD is a true disease, this clinician asks, why do we only suspect it in classrooms?

Neurological Approaches to ADHD

The most significant point of difference between psychodynamic and neurological stances toward ADHD concerns the perceived essence of hyperactivity, impulsivity, and inattention. As we shall see, neurology reduces ADHD-like symptoms to biological processes, streamlining the way ADHD is diagnosed and simultaneously invalidating psychodynamic reasoning. The belief in the effectiveness of amphetamine-based medications remains a key separation between psychodynamic perspectives and neurology. The reported effects of such medications validate neurology's complex nomenclature, ratifying biologically oriented clinical practices while providing a window into the true "soul" of the ADHD child—a neurologically challenged soul where deviant behavior is attributed to a nonhuman agent.

Neurology's Critique of the Psychodynamic View of ADHD

Authors who contribute to the modern psychodynamic discussion of ADHD profess two propositions that pull their audiences in contradictory directions: (1) ADHD is a biological reality; (2) ADHD is a misunderstood, overly diagnosed social construct. As Lawrence Diller (1998, 82) states:

> There is some evidence that children identified as ADD at age three or four continued to show problems later in childhood; this suggests that ADD is a "stable" characteristic. . . . However, I'm not so sure that biologically driven behavior is the only problem in this scenario; sometimes being labeled as having a "disorder" can contribute to ongoing negative behaviors.

From a sociological angle, Diller claims that there are outside forces—labeling agents perhaps as powerful as the actual biological phenomenon of ADHD—that contribute to the behavioral problems associated with it. The bona fide case of ADHD then, has organic and social causes. Critics of this perspective claim it leaves too many unanswered questions about the nature of ADHD, and allows too many ADHD children to fall through the psychodynamic cracks, so to speak. Such a position, they argue, prevents the formation of a universal discussion of ADHD and a universal treatment of the disorder.

Discussions of the etiology of ADHD in terms of family dynamics and the consequent promotion of psychotherapy as a crucial form of ADHD treatment have been, and continue to be, under considerable attack. Perspectives depicting ADHD as a pure neurological entity seek a unified theory about the causes of the disorder. Such a perspective first attempts to provide a solid position on the etiology of ADHD and second, champions incontrovertibly effective pharmacological treatment.

The strictly physiological perspective on ADHD championed by neurologists relegates children with ADHD-like symptoms into uncharted areas of pathology. According to this perspective, these children exhibit "soft" neurologic signs (Bray 1969, 14) that are not clearly identifiable within the available conceptual schemes in neurology. For example, disease categories such as the *aphasias*, which denote disturbance in language ability, the *apraxias*, which affect the ability to carry out motor activity and contain focused attention, and the *agnosias*, which involve strong disturbances in recognition, prove inadequate in accounting for this rather nebulous childhood malady (Ford 1948). There are two major reasons for this inadequacy. First, the aforementioned disease categories and numerous others all directly implicate organic lesions, commonly attributable to localized regions of the brain. For ADHD, there is no discernible lesion to be held accountable. Second, such ailments are given empirical credibility through their representation in tests that hone in on the specific nature of the neurological impairment. The Bender-Gestalt test, for example, proves adequate in discovering children with language impairment, as in the case of a form of *aphasia*, but fails miserably in validating an ADHD diagnosis. We are left, then, with a mode of reverse engineering not uncommon to modern neurology and the clinicians who stay true to the aims of the neurological enterprise: the collection of symptoms to be diagnosed as ADHD are better understood if treated first and analyzed later.

Addressing the Work of Paul Wender

Paul Wender (1971), a strict adherent to the neurological perspective to-ward ADHD and its conceptual precursors, and a staunch critic of psychodynamic stances toward the disorder, has been the most signifi-cant researcher in the effort to summarize this litany of childhood behav-ioral problems under a single medical diagnosis. Though minimal brain dysfunction (MBD) was adopted as the official diagnosis of impulsive and disruptive childhood behavior by the United States Public Health Service (USPHS) in 1966 (Conrad 1975), there remained a barrage of other clinical terms describing similar collections of symptoms. Arguing from a neurological stance, Wender expressed a strong desire to unify the nomenclature that describes the symptoms of impulsivity, hyperkinesis, and the like in children. Wender is the first to ask the medical community to abandon what he termed to be the outdated nomenclature of "minimal brain damage," "minimal cerebral palsy," "minimal cerebral dysfunc-tion," "maturational lag," "post-encephalitic disorder" and universally adopt the term "minimal brain dysfunction" (Wender 1971, 2).

The perspectives regarding the childhood difficulties of impulsivity and hyperkinesis that were purported by Paul Wender, Leon Eisenberg, and others, gained some universality in the psychiatric community (Con-rad 1976). By the mid-1970s, MBD became the dominant way both cli-nicians and researchers characterized such childhood problems. The ter-minology of MBD was deemed appropriate for a neurological perspec-tive on childhood behavior that was unconventional and anti-institutional and yet not so deviant that it warranted a more serious sounding diagnos-tic category. MBD described a condition in children that implicated physiological malfunction (e.g., "brain dysfunction"), and yet through the use of the word "minimal," this condition was described as mild enough to be effectively treated. In spite of the fact that their problematic behaviors were perceived to be a result of a neurological impairment, children diagnosed with MBD were promised that they could be reinte-grated into conventional living through treatment with appropriate medi-cation. MBD was to be taken seriously—it was a collection of symptoms worthy of a medical diagnosis—but it was also fixable. In keeping with the same reasoning that typified the discussion of moral imbecility and the psychiatric sequelae of *encephalitis lethargica*, MBD described anti-institutional childhood behavior, but the diagnosis of MBD furthered these discussions by being inextricably linked to specific methods of drug treatment.

Due in part to pressures outside the medical establishment, MBD eventually fell out of favor with those in clinical circles (Kessler 1980). The main reason for this was the stigmatizing effects of the words "brain dysfunction," primarily that they demarcated children with impulsivity and attention problems as having some kind of brain *damage*—a condition understood to be irreparable. Furthermore, the American Psychiatric Association never officially adopted minimal brain dysfunction as a diagnostic category. Though not widely used in clinical circles, the APA's 1968 *Diagnostic and Statistical Manual of Mental Disorders,* second edition (*DSM II*) avoided the language of "brain damage" and "dysfunction" and adopted the phrase, "hyperkinetic reaction of childhood" (50). Summarized in a single paragraph,[3] "hyperkinetic reaction of childhood" represented yet another interpretation of such childhood difficulties and was far from universally adopted by clinicians and researchers. By the time *DSM III* was published in 1980, the APA's nomenclature, not that of the USPHS, had become the dominant way to interpret these childhood behavioral problems. Immensely popular with clinicians (see Kirk and Kutchins 1992), *DSM III* was the first of the manuals to include a discussion of childhood problems of inattention in addition to hyperactive symptoms (Breggin 1998). *DSM III* described a condition called attention deficit disorder, beginning the now popularized acronym ADD. Subsequent neurological theories that attempted to link physiological mechanisms of attention and overactivity prompted the APA to reformulate the typology for both childhood inattention and hyperactivity. The term *Attention Deficit-Hyperactivity Disorder* (*ADHD*) combined both ADD and hyperkinesis into one disease category and was included in the publication of the *Diagnostic and Statistical Manual of Mental Disorders,* third edition, revised (*DSM III-R*) in 1987. ADHD denoted the neurological dominance of the discussion of such childhood problems, particularly that the same neurological problem could manifest itself in different ways with different children. A case of ADHD might be characterized by inattentiveness, hyperactivity, or a combination of these.

Currently, according to the APA's (1994) *DSM IV* criteria, ADHD is part of a class of mental disorders that are "Usually First Diagnosed in Infancy, Childhood, or Adolescence" and may be diagnosed if certain conditions are met in a clinical assessment. These conditions are represented by five major criteria, listed A through E (APA 1994, 83-5). Within criterion A we see the symptoms that are most typically attributed to popular notions of ADHD and are the major basis for providing ADHD diagnoses. Criterion A is divided into symptoms of "inattention" (criterion A1)[4] and "hyperactivity-impulsivity" (criterion A2),[5] in which nine types of symptoms are described for each.

In diagnosing symptoms in criterion A1 and/or A2, *DSM IV* recommends that a positive diagnosis be made if at least six of the symptoms from either or both of these criteria "have persisted for at least six months to a degree that is maladaptive and inconsistent with developmental level" (83-4). Based upon the assessments made by a clinician, the type of ADHD diagnosed may be placed within one of three categories. These are: (1) "Attention-Deficit/Hyperactivity Disorder, Combined Type" (*DSM IV* code 314.01), in which both criteria A1 and A2 (that is, at least six symptoms from each) are met for at least six months; (2) "Attention-Deficit/Hyperactivity Disorder, Predominantly Inattentive Type" (*DSM IV* code 314.00), in which criterion A1 is met; and (3) "Attention-Deficit/Hyperactivity Disorder, Predominantly Hyperactive-Impulsive Type" (*DSM IV* code 314.01). ADHD, then, can manifest itself in various forms and in varying intensities of two different types of problem behavior, according to the APA. The current *DSM IV* criteria for ADHD unify two rather disparate types of behavior—one characterized by extroversion, the other by introversion—into a single, subdivided disease category.

Neurologically Oriented Clinicians and the "Straightforward" Case of ADHD

As their clinical approach to ADHD resonates with a neurological stance, pediatricians and general practitioners take a relatively short time in diagnosing ADHD when compared to their psychodynamically oriented counterparts. Exemplifying this, one pediatrician explains that diagnosing a case of ADHD may take "one hour if it's straightforward... I'll look at a Conners[6] if the child has already been given that test" (pediatrician, age forty-seven). In the "straightforward" case of ADHD, the time to provide a diagnosis and prescribe treatment—usually medication—is contained within the space of a doctor visit lasting anywhere from thirty to sixty minutes. The straightforward case of ADHD clarifies the distinction between "hard-wired" ADHD and other psychological problems that may impede a clear and rapid diagnosis. Reflecting neurology's pointed criticisms of psychodynamic approaches to ADHD, such clinicians concur that a proper diagnosis should not become bogged down in irrelevant psychological problems. As one pediatrician explains: "Our job is to address a problem with the brain, not to restructure everything a child does."

Clinicians who use a regimented amount of time to diagnose a case of ADHD often claim to have considerable information before seeing the suspected child. Prior to their clinical visit, it is common for children and parents to have already completed questionnaires or Conners Scales in other locations, most often in the office of a school nurse or school psychologist. In such cases, which make up the bulk of patients of neurologically oriented clinicians, the results of diagnostic tests such as the Conners Scale are already provided to clinicians prior to a formal interview with a child—a situation that emphasizes the role of nonclinical agents in medically labeling ADHD children. Clearly, one of the functions of the Conners Scale is to expand the diagnostic abilities of nonclinical parties. As one clinician states: "It always helps if they do a lot of the work for us, so that when we're in here (referring to the clinic) we can get down to the real problem. It's just a smarter way to do things" (general practitioner, age fifty-five). Ideally, the scale provides a means to compiling data that could later be formally analyzed by a clinician. In its practical application, however, clinicians state that much of the analyses of Conners Scales had occurred prior to a clinical visit. The diagnosis of ADHD is provided more quickly because clinicians examine the results of a diagnostic test rather than taking time to administer it themselves.

The Unquestioning Use of *DSM IV*

In contrast to respondents who either had reservations about *DSM IV*'s ability to adequately describe ADHD or questioned its specific language, some clinicians argue that *DSM IV* is integral in providing a diagnosis of ADHD. Some adapted *DSM IV* criteria to questionnaires that are commonly filled out by their patients. As one pediatrician explains, "We give them a sheet with those criteria to fill out in the waiting room. I let my secretary know what it may be and she gets it ready for them." Another physician explains that using the *DSM IV* is very important in keeping him focused on what he is treating: "The *DSM* gives me my box to work within. I use it to tell me the boundaries of the person's problem. If they fall too far outside that or don't fit into it at all, I may recommend a bigger psychiatric evaluation" (general practitioner, age fifty-five). In this case, *DSM IV* is presented as a crucial tool of evaluation, providing the boundaries for further assessment.

The "Disease Process" Narrative of ADHD

Before exploring clinicians' accounts of the disease process of ADHD, it is important to return to the broader discussion of neurological discourse.

As a champion of the cause of unifying what was at that time called MBD, Paul Wender (1971) argued that MBD was plainly misunderstood within the psychodynamic community. According to Wender, psycho-dynamic interpretations of MBD failed to address an "underlying disease process" (Wender 1971, 83). Wender further argued that the continuing psychodynamic studies of MBD that examine constantly changing mani-festations of the same neurological pathology rather than the organic trauma itself were clinically useless. Due to the large variability in the symptoms of this condition, Wender claimed, psychologists and psycho-analysts provided a chaotic myriad of causes and treatments of these symptoms. They were lost in the symptoms, and psychotherapy provided mere "Band-Aids" for a more complex phenomenon. As Wender argued, over time, the inadequacy of psychodynamic treatments became easier to assert as people who exhibited MBD symptoms as children continued to struggle into adulthood (Wender 1971, 84). From Wender's view, people do not grow out of MBD. This is not because psychotherapy is not re-fined or insightful enough but because the underlying disease remains untreated.

In criticizing Phyllis Greenacre's work, Wender contended that psy-chological perspectives of MBD that analyze nonphysiological influ-ences upon the child's behavior (i.e., the family) are predisposed to an examination of "secondary reactions" to the syndrome (Wender 1971, 82). Wender contrasts these secondary reactions with the less-understood primary reactions to the disorder. The primary reactions are directly linked to the physiology of MBD and include "decrease in the experience of pleasure or pain," "poorly modulated activation" (being overreactive to stress), "generally high level of activation" (hyperactivity), and "ex-troversion" (social aggression) (Wender 1971, 136-41). The secondary reactions, which compose the bulk of data for psychological studies, in-clude "narcissism," "depression," and "immaturity" (Wender 1971, 141-51).

Wender argued that psychologists often interpreted such secondary reactions as coming from "events" in the child's life rather than neurological difficulties. These events, as psychologists understood them, were believed to be directly linked to the anxiety experienced by children as it arose from their inability to succeed in the world. Organically disordered children react violently to a world they do not understand. A cycle of hostility is then perceived to take place involving children and their immediate environment, making up "the events" clinicians choose to fruitlessly unravel. The perception is that an initial difficulty or anxiety would become greatly exacerbated by the reactions of others toward the child. The physiological difficulty becomes far less significant than the damaging patterns children and their families incorporate into daily life. An example of the relationship between organic brain trauma, anxiety, and consequent behavior can be found most commonly in schools. A student who has a physical incapacity to perform well in school might exhibit moderate to severe disciplinary problems due to continued frustration with that environment. Proponents of a psychodynamic view contend that the causes of these problems are social rather than neurological.

Wender and others who argued from a neurological stance contended that anxiety was very difficult to measure empirically. Moreover, to say that anxiety was a disabling agent for an MBD child was equally questionable. Wender provides two grounds for this assertion: (1) in "pure cases" of MBD the conditions that psychologists call anxiety are difficult if not impossible to find; and (2) the history of studying childhood anxiety has been tainted by samples of children with a variety of different mental disorders—schizophrenia, for example—rather than cases whose symptoms specifically implicated MBD (Wender 1971, 146-7).

Wender argued that MBD should be understood as a syndrome with a complex of symptoms rather than a disorder with a specific set of symptoms (Wender 1971, 135). The variations in symptoms could, in effect, be attributable to subtypes, and MBD may adequately become the rubric under which related pathologies would be categorized. A clinician might diagnose MBD of a hyperkinetic type, or another with a more cognitive manifestation, for example. Regardless of subtype, and Wender hypothesized that there were many, the proponents of neurology argued that the basics of MBD could be understood through a greater accumulation of knowledge about the chemical structure of the brain. The most important means to acquiring this knowledge was the chemical treatment of MBD symptoms. A child's reaction to medication, such as Ritalin, continues to be seen as an inductive tool to ascertain the physical condition of the child. Through the administration of medicines, to which children's responses are monitored, dosages altered, and medicine type changed, a thorough neurological picture of the child's difficulty becomes visible, they argued.[7]

To bring this neurological discussion into a contemporary light, we must make mention of Russell Barkley (1991, 1997), who has been at the forefront of the neurological perspective on ADHD and whose ideas have formulated the bulk of the discussion of ADHD in popular media.[8] His work has been pivotal in framing the relationship between ADHD and nerve cell receptor site abnormalities, with a specific focus on the connection between the neurotransmitter dopamine and the ability to resist impulses. Dopamine, it is argued, is a chemical that regulates emotion and movement. A faulty receptor site for dopamine can fail to register incoming dopamine signals from another neuron. A dopamine transporter is said to reclaim the unused dopamine before the receptor can receive it. Hence, not enough dopamine travels appropriately through the nerve fibers. Without enough transference of this neurotransmitter, ADHD children are supposedly unable to inhibit emotional and physical responses to outside stimuli. Popular accounts of ADHD are heavily influenced by this neurological discourse. Using the work of Barkley, a *U.S. News and World Report* article, for example, summarized the condition of ADHD in neurological terms, yet the discussion was simplified enough to be digestible by a lay audience (Brink 1998).

Clinicians Describing Dopamine Disregulation/Brain Underactivation as a Cause of ADHD

Though there is no exam that specifically describes ADHD, some of the common narrative about the cause of this disorder invokes neurological dysfunction, often attributable to brain underactivation and a problem with the regulation of dopamine (Barkley 1997, Fuster 1997). As one clinician describes:

> There's an underactivation in the prefrontal cortex, primarily with the dopaminergic pathways that are not being activated correctly. There is less ability to regulate oneself from this. Executive functions are asleep at the switch. Stimulant medication may stimulate activity in that center (psychiatrist, age forty-seven).

Another respondent links dopamine disregulation to specific regions of the brain:

> The frontal region controls impulses, gives us social inhibi-
> tion. We can see that kids with ADHD don't have this area of
> the brain activated as well. . . . Ritalin is a dopamine stimulant
> that activates this part of the brain. It's like taking insulin if
> you're diabetic. The body isn't circulating a chemical prop-
> erly, so drugs like Ritalin make an abnormal situation normal
> (pediatrician, age forty-two).

These two excerpts contain three propositions that strongly represent the bulk of responses that addressed the issue of dopamine disregulation and brain underactivation.

First, there is the description of the ADHD child's brain as underacti-vated. This condition, described very well in lay person's terms by Gabor Mate (2000, 40-1), is the root of the "ADHD paradox." Common sense might conclude that ADHD children exhibiting hyperactivity and an in-ability to focus on important tasks suffer from an *over*-activation of the brain. With the case of ADHD, the reverse is supposedly true. Certain mechanisms within the brain that facilitate focus and social restraint are argued to not be adequately activated.

Second, ADHD symptoms are seemingly linked to underactivation in a particular region of the brain: the frontal lobe, and more specifically, the prefrontal cortex. Within the ADHD brain, dopaminergic pathways are not operating to full capacity; hence, the neurotransmitter dopamine is argued to be greatly reduced. As mentioned, dopamine is the neuro-transmitter most commonly linked to the exercise of social restraint. Less dopamine circulating throughout the frontal lobe equates to less inhibi-tion. Inhibition, in this sense, keeps a child on task by effectively staving off interest in distractions. A child with normal brain activation and nor-mal levels of inhibition can demonstrate restraint in negotiating between the tasks at hand and distractions, such as peripheral sounds, friends making funny faces, or the internal desire to get out of one's seat and run about the classroom. In addition, the prefrontal cortex is also strongly associated with metacognition and self-awareness. As one clinician states, in a "normal" brain the "executive functions" are intact, enabling a normal amount of awareness about one's own thinking and how one's behavior affects other people. ADHD children are described as very lim-ited in this capacity. Because the prefrontal cortex lacks adequate stimu-lation, such children are not able to take a reflective stance toward their patterns of thinking or their behavior. They act out because "they have to."

The third proposition concerns the effect of stimulant medication upon the ADHD brain. Through PET scans, it has been demonstrated that stimulants such as Ritalin increase the circulation of dopamine in the frontal region of the brain and consequently enhance an ADHD child's ability for restraint and task-oriented behavior. Supposedly, such medication rectifies an abnormal situation by increasing dopamine levels comparably to those in the "normal" population.

The ADHD Science War

As it clearly is the dominant voice in both academic and popular media, and given the fact that the primary treatment for ADHD has shifted almost entirely towards medication, it may easily be argued that the neurological perspective on ADHD, despite the diagnostic uncertainty that surrounds the disorder, is the dominant lens through which ADHD is understood. It is important to address why the neurological perspective on ADHD has gained practical dominance and also include the voices of skepticism that linger despite this.

Neurology's scientific "evidence" of the causes and presence of ADHD derives technical support from diagnostic devices that are directly linked to the criteria for ADHD. This represents a significant point of departure for neurologists in comparison to their psychodynamic counterparts. As they are largely inductive in nature, psychodynamic methods of diagnosing and treating ADHD-like symptoms fail to consistently implicate a singular disease process. As asserted by Wender (1971), it is widely believed in neurological circles that understandings of ADHD symptoms that ignore neurology become hopelessly intertwined with a melange of symptoms and therefore fail to address an essential organic condition.

Two of the most popular diagnostic technologies for ADHD include the aforementioned Conners Scale and Positron Emission Tomography (PET) scans. PET scans of the brain begin by having a patient swallow a small amount of radioactive glucose that makes its way into the circulatory system of the brain and becomes visible through electromagnetic scanning. By charting where the glucose can be seen, researchers claim that they find fundamental differences in the brains of patients with ADHD and patients without the disorder. The contention is that patients diagnosed with ADHD have less of the glucose visible in specific regions of the brain that enable impulse inhibition and the discrimination between important and unimportant stimuli. These differences in brain structure are argued to cause an underactivation in the brain's frontal lobe, which in turn causes distractibility and erratic behavior (Mataro 1997, Matthys et al. 1999). Furthermore, researchers argue that medication therapy restores the frontal lobe to a normal level of activation, which can apparently be seen in the increased amounts of radioactive glucose in subsequent PET scans (Barkley 1997).

PET scans have been subject to considerable criticism, particularly that the results of such exams where ADHD is concerned centers on patients who have already been prescribed stimulant medication (Breggin 1998) and also that the interpretation of PET scans is highly unreliable (Walker 1998). Critics assert that test groups who comprise the bulk of subjects for PET scans have previously been diagnosed with ADHD and have often already begun taking drugs such as Cylert, Dexedrine, and Ritalin. Hence, it is argued that the results of PET scans validate the opinions of those who are opposed to the ADHD diagnosis as such scans reveal the brain-altering effects of Ritalin rather than an inherent brain structure abnormality. In addition, it is asserted that electrochemical reactions in the brain are naturally volatile, subject to emotional states and levels of physical stress. Because of this, it is argued that the brain profiles of children who undergo PET scans may vary from day to day, even from moment to moment. In sum, ADHD skeptics argue that those who believe in the existence of ADHD use the largely ambiguous results of PET scans for their own ideological aims.

The response to such criticism can be seen in the ever expanding quest for adequate methods of ADHD diagnosis. For example, one experimental test, the optical tracking and attention test (OPTax), is the current pinnacle of neurology's quest to definitively detect the presence of ADHD. Invented by Harvard University psychiatrist Martin Teicher, this test involves children tracking moving targets on a computer screen and monitors the children's success in responding to the targets. As Richard Wronski (2001) states in a *Chicago Tribune* article: "During the 15 minute OPTax test, the child sits before a computer screen and is challenged to respond to the appearance of moving stars. The speed and accuracy of the child's responses provide data on attentiveness and impulsiveness." While the child is responding to the stars moving on the computer screen, an infrared camera follows a marker that has been placed on the back of the child's head. Throughout its duration the OPTax exam meticulously monitors and tallies every minute fidget a child makes. The data collected from the OPTax test are compared with scores from thousands of other children. From these scores, a continuum of hyperactivity and/or inattention is constructed and becomes the standard by which children who take the OPTax are assessed.

The search for the essence of ADHD is characterized by ever advancing technology—Connors Scales, PET scans, OPTax exams, and so on—but, as numerous critics convey, the results of this quest leave considerable doubt. Neurologically minded ADHD researchers claim that the disease process of ADHD is clear and that the results of a PET scan "discover" ADHD in the same fashion as diabetes or cancer. However, when the findings of neurology are placed within the context of the historical and contemporary ambiguity surrounding ADHD, the claim that the "essence" of ADHD has been uncovered appears hopeful at best, ideological at worst. Until there is an incontrovertible method for diagnosing ADHD, this debate will continue, and justifiably so. However, given the vast number of children who are diagnosed with ADHD and taking medication, and given the relative absence of psychotherapy for the ADHD-diagnosed, we must conclude that neurology reigns supreme, at least for now.

In the face of such an onslaught of technical explorations of ADHD, psychodynamic perspectives struggle with how they will account for and treat the disorder. Through its examinations and documentation measures, neurology offers a biological explanation that distinguishes between the "maladjusted" child and the ADHD child. Psychodynamic nomenclature cannot capture this distinction. The psychodynamic perspective wallows in the ambiguities that its discourse describes: an ADHD child may or may not have organic brain damage, may or may not need extensive therapy, may or may not need to be medicated. From the perspective of neurology, these become nonissues once a positive diagnosis of ADHD is made. If a child responds positively to the administration of a medication, the diagnosis is validated.

The contemporary, neurological account of ADHD is clearly an example of psychiatry "re-biologizing itself," denoting the increasing push in psychiatry to realign itself with the natural sciences and return to the time before the psychoanalytic "mental hygiene" movement (Young 1995, 270). The acronym "ADHD" represents the perspective of neurology, its wide recognition reflecting neurology's substantial influence. From Michel Foucault's (1978, 101-2) perspective, ADHD may be said to represent a moment of dominance within the field of "force relations," in which discourses strategize to lay claim to a particular object of knowledge, which are realized simultaneously with the deployment of power. As Foucault (1978) proposes: "the rationality of power is characterized by tactics which, becoming connected to one another, attracting and propagating one another, but finding their base of support and their condition elsewhere, end by forming comprehensive systems" (95). When we think we have attained knowledge about ADHD, we are subject to a relation of power. This moment of knowing designates one narrative's temporary dominance over another. For Foucault, the objects that are constructed by these discourses and their proponents are constantly in flux: "ADHD Regimes" have been created but are not entirely monolithic.

Notes

1. The discussion of "nipping the illness in the bud" is still prevalent in today's discussion of ADHD. Numerous studies have been published that argue that there is a relationship between childhood ADHD and later antisocial mental disorders more associated with teenagers and adults. For example, it has been argued that there is a high coincidence (or "comorbidity" in psychiatric terms) of ADHD with Conduct Disorder and Oppositional Defiant Disorder (ODD) as ADHD children grow older (Baving et al. 1999). Though the rates vary, some studies have shown comorbidity rates to be as high as 93 percent in community-based samples (Jensen and Cantwell 1997). The levels of comorbidity are argued to have both organic and social causes. Some researchers argue that the comorbidity of Conduct Disorder and ODD with ADHD is simply due to abnormalities in brain function (Matthys et al. 1999), but others lean more toward an interpretation favoring social maladjustment, or "psychosocial" difficulties due to early ADHD (Barkley et al. 1993). Regardless of the various arguments that depict the reasons for this comorbidity, current clinical discussions contend that ADHD symptoms must be addressed before the condition solidifies and becomes "too late" for the child.

2. It is also relevant that Freud's patient was female. Modern scientific narrative about ADHD, though still "in progress" regarding gender, contends that girls have different electroencephalographic activity from boys, prompting them to exhibit more inattentive types of behavior (see Baving et al. 1999).

3. It is clear from this discussion that the APA saw a vast difference between psychodynamic and physiological reasons for hyperkinetic phenomena in children. As *DSM II* states: "If this behavior is caused by organic brain damage, it

should be diagnosed under the appropriate non-psychotic *organic brain syndrome*" (50; emphasis in original).

4. The nine symptoms of inattention are: "a) often fails to give close attention to details or makes careless mistakes in schoolwork, work, or other activities; b) often has difficulty sustaining attention in tasks or play activities; c) often does not seem to listen when spoken to directly; d) often does not follow through on instructions and fails to finish schoolwork, chores, or duties in the workplace (not due to oppositional behavior, or failure to understand directions); f) often avoids, dislikes, or is reluctant to engage in tasks that require sustained mental effort (such as schoolwork or homework); g) often loses things necessary for tasks or activities (e.g., toys, school assignments, pencils, books, or tools); h) is often distracted by outside stimuli; i) is often forgetful in daily activities" (83-4).

5. For hyperactivity-impulsivity, the symptoms are "a) often fidgets with hands or squirms in seat; b) often leaves seat in classroom or in other situations in which remaining seated is expected; c) often runs about or climbs excessively in situations in which it is inappropriate (in adolescents or adults, may be limited to subjective feelings of restlessness); d) often has difficulty playing or engaging in leisure activities quietly; e) is often "on the go," or often acts as if "driven by a motor"; f) often talks excessively; g) often blurts out answers before questions have been completed; h) often has difficulty awaiting turn; i) often interrupts or intrudes on others (e.g., butts into conversations or games)" (84).

6. The Conners Rating Scale (CRS) was originated by C. Keith Conners (1969) and has become the most utilized method of trying to diagnose ADHD and other problem childhood behavior. This scale, originally intended to provide a basis for prescribing children stimulant medication, has gone through many revisions in its thirty-year-plus history. Currently, it follows *DSM IV* guidelines to try and tease out problem childhood behavior. In the long version of the forms (there are forms for teachers and parents, both of which are gender-specific), a white to red shading scheme reveals the possible presence of a *DSM IV* diagnosis. If the score falls within the red color, the clinician may be alerted to a possible disorder. There is also a Conners "Self Report" that children themselves fill out.

7. Clinicians' accounts of the administration of medications will be addressed at length in chapter 4.

8. For other popular accounts of ADHD that are sympathetic to a neurological perspective on ADHD see *USA Today*, August 11, 2003, 7d; *Business Week*, April 14, 2003, 86-8; *Business Week*, Nov. 22, 1999, 70; *The Clearing House*, September-October 1999, 43; *Newsweek*, December 7, 1999, 60; *Runner's World*, July 1999, 84. *Time*, November 30, 1998, 86-92; *U.S. News and World Report*, December 27, 1999, 12.

Chapter Four

Clinicians as the Mediators of ADHD Suspicion and Treatment

Regardless of whether they adopt a psychodynamic, neurological, or some other approach to ADHD, clinicians are regarded as "experts" on the disorder. Because of this, clinicians represent the medium between a child suspected of having ADHD and the diagnosis and treatment plan afforded to such a child. In addressing from where or from whom they usually hear the first suspicions of a child possibly having ADHD, clinicians' experiences highlight the connections between different parties during the process of diagnosis and treatment and also reveal the motivations for people to approach them with such suspicion. As clinicians explain in some detail how they are approached, and what they feel are some of the motivating factors behind being approached, they give specific examples of how lay people attempt to resolve childhood struggles through a formal diagnostic process.

This chapter will first explore how clinicians are approached with a "possible" case of ADHD. ADHD suspicions, which are garnered primarily in the school, are seen by some clinicians as an aid in ADHD diagnoses, whereas other clinicians regard the informal assessments made in schools as an encroachment upon their own professional obligations. As many clinicians contend, the school's main intention in approaching them is to get a child on medication. Second, this chapter will explore the treatment protocols that are followed after a suspected ADHD case is brought to clinicians. This discussion further demonstrates the rift between psychodynamic and neurological approaches to ADHD. What I illustrate through analyses of literature and clinicians' own accounts is that pharmacological approaches to ADHD have been and continue to be the subject of considerable ambivalence.

Clinician Interactions with School Representatives

Regardless of their stance towards the causes and treatment of ADHD, clinicians almost universally convey that intervention from school authorities is the major action that moves a suspected case of ADHD into a formal clinical environment. The consistent discussion of schools reveals that there is an institutionally specific context for the suspicion of ADHD. And, as will be shown in subsequent chapters, this is corroborated by parents who almost universally invoke the school as a source of struggle that precipitated suspicions of ADHD and a subsequent visit to some type of clinical expert.

Institutional locations of suspicion are consistent with the very early discussion of ADHD symptoms implicit in the work on the psychological sequelae of *encephalitis lethargica* by Kennedy (1924), Ebaugh (1923), Stryker (1925), and others discussed in chapter 2. The historical depiction of ADHD symptoms implicated problems in institutional contexts, the school chief among them. As I will discuss later in this chapter, the institution of education was a point of interest in experiments with the first trials of unruly children taking Benzedrine in 1937, in which it was concluded that children who took the drug began making dramatic improvements in both comprehension of and enthusiasm for schoolwork. These and other studies illustrate that problems in school have been historically seen as indicative of severe social maladjustment, and improvement in school performance is equated to "appropriate" social behavior.

We understand the desires of an institution by its representatives. Therefore, if we are to understand the situation of a to-be-diagnosed case of ADHD, we need to see how these institutional representatives interact with formal mechanisms of diagnosis and treatment. For example, clinicians commonly attribute parents' solicitation of a formal ADHD assessment for their children to pressure from their child's school. As one pediatrician states: "They [parents] approach me after having some problems with the school. They say 'The teacher has some real problems with my kid and wanted me to have him assessed.'" Parents are not discussed as parties owning sole agency in bringing their children to be formally diagnosed but rather as arriving at the clinician's office with an incentive from the school. In this capacity, parents represent the desires of the institution of education. In discussing the school's role in presenting a possible case of ADHD to a formal clinical realm, the interviews reveal that schools, or at least the element of schools that is the most antagonistic toward unruly children, are integral in drawing attention to such children. Common representatives in this regard are school counselors and teachers, whom many clinicians regard as crucial in suspecting ADHD and in providing a preliminary diagnosis of the disorder. Due to this, clinicians often see themselves as people who *confirm* an ADHD diagnosis, rather than originate or discover one. One pediatrician with fifteen years of experience in treating ADHD states: "A majority of the referrals come from the schools. The teacher will say they need to get a kid assessed. There are times when they say, 'We have an ADD here.'" Another clinician put the experience this way:

> The child is most often referred to me by the school. I usually talk to a guidance counselor or a resource teacher or something like that. The school tends to diagnose these kids prior to them coming to me. They are sent to me for a reason and that's medication. The school doesn't usually directly confront the parents and tell them to go to the doctor and get some pills to fix their kid. They come to me first, but they want me to refer them to a doctor for the meds (family therapist, age fifty-two).

Recalling clinicians who merely "collect information," ADHD assessments given at school clearly lessen clinicians' own diagnostic role. Further, many clinicians contend that medications are the underlying motivation for school authorities to approach them with suspicions of a child's having ADHD. Serving as gatekeepers between schools and the authority to prescribe medications, clinicians often cast themselves as a means to an end. These "ends" include a change in the child's social and/or academic behavior, believed to be achievable through stimulant medication. In doing clinical assessments of a "probable" ADHD case as decreed by a school, clinicians claim there is a pressure to confirm these suspicions and start the process of administering medication: "I think, ultimately the school knows what they want. It's really about a behavioral problem they want solved, and they know that the best way to fix it is through meds. ...I make the decision, but I'm well aware of what decision they would like me to make" (psychiatrist, age forty-eight). It is also argued that this type of involvement with a case of ADHD makes the school's intervention less intrusive. Instead of directly recommending that parents place their children on Ritalin, schools may encourage an assessment by a professional, such as a family therapist, to confirm the abnormalcy of a child's behavior and prompt a physician referral.

For many clinicians, the role school authorities play in suspecting ADHD is considered an integral aspect of the diagnosis process: "This is a disorder that is usually first discovered in the school, and that's one of the reasons why teachers need to gain more awareness of this disorder, know what to look for" (clinical psychologist, age thirty-nine). Many clinicians state that more needs to be done in order for schools to accurately assess the possible presence of ADHD. Hence, a major theme mentioned in the interviews concerns the need to educate teachers on the ADHD diagnosis and help them recognize the disorder in their students. This perceived need to make teachers understand more about ADHD is directed at both classroom and administrative levels. As one clinician states:

> Well, some teachers think that it's not real. We need to keep trying to educate teachers that ADHD is very real. It's not recognized as an LD [learning disability]. You've got these kids in classes who are 'winging it' and because ADHD is not recognized, they have no real way out (psychiatrist, age forty-seven).

Clinicians also express the need for teachers to also adjust how they react to ADHD behaviors:

> It's important for teachers to ID [identify] the kids who may be at risk. They have to learn more about the disorder for that to occur. If you don't know what to look for, then you won't find it. Teachers spend all this time punishing kids who are acting out, but they never stop to think 'Hey, I wonder if this kid might have something really wrong here' (pediatrician, age forty-seven).

There is a relationship between education about ADHD and an increase in the ability to profile the disorder, it is argued. That is, the connection between knowledge of ADHD and the recognition of it exemplifies the process of framing deviant classroom behavior as a medical problem. Through sensitizing teachers to the condition of ADHD, a more specific deviance label can be applied, rather than those that describe "slow" or "lazy" students.

In conjunction with statements that teachers need to have an increased awareness of the symptoms of ADHD, clinicians also argue that teachers need to tailor their reactions to these children. As one clinician states:

"Teachers, for whatever reason, might not have the resources or the skills. They get into this pejorative stance, which really only rationalizes their frustration" (clinical psychologist, age forty-five). Because ADHD children are perceived by some clinicians to be neurologically different, the normal standards for judging these children's misbehavior falter. As they largely perceive ADHD-related behavior as outside of a child's control, clinicians argue that teachers' reactions to such children should avoid punitive stances that in the instance of a "normal," unruly and academically/socially challenged child might be appropriate. To punish ADHD children for their behavior through detention or the removal of privileges is perceived as an act of ignorance.

Disputed Territory: Professional Conflict between Clinicians and Teachers

In contrast to those clinicians stating that teachers need to become better at recognizing ADHD and advance their involvement in diagnosing it, some clinicians describe teachers as becoming too involved in the suspicion and diagnosis process: "First of all, teachers are not therapists. Their job is to teach, not to start labeling kids as having some kind of mental disorder when it may be their fault in the first place. Sure, they need to be aware, but they have to look at their part in things" (family therapist, age fifty-two). And another clinician: "I think educators spend a lot of their time trying to confirm that a kid may have ADHD, when they aren't necessarily qualified to offer that kind of information. Teachers aren't doctors and I don't think they should be recommending that parents put their children on medication" (pediatrician, age fifty-seven).

Teachers' hybridized pedagogical and clinical role with respect to ADHD places them in a position in which their diagnostic prowess is viewed as a professional encroachment, according to some clinicians. The difference between informally suspecting a child and formally declaring his/her condition is argued to represent the necessary distinction between educational and clinical contexts. To not honor this distinction or to turn the classroom into a "semi-official clinic," according to some clinicians, creates the dangerous possibility of misdiagnoses. It is also claimed that teachers' own suspicions of children may be an indirect way of avoiding their own responsibilities, shuffling their professional problems (e.g., students who are disruptive and academically slow) onto the backs of clinicians. By arguing that teachers avert their gaze from "their part in things" and label children as having ADHD, clinicians claim that teachers begin an unjustified labeling process in which problem behaviors are attributed to a mental disorder rather than the environment that causes or exacerbates those problem behaviors. By beginning the process of labeling a child, it is argued, the institution of education never reflects upon its own role in the child's difficulties.

The professional antagonism between clinicians and teachers illustrates the tremendous influx of ADHD knowledge into classrooms in recent years and reflects the defense of established realms of clinical expertise. It is an example of the vicissitudes of the micro-politics of trouble (Emerson and Messinger 1977), in which the path to medicalizing behavior may be complicated by the struggle over definitions of profession and the rights to knowledge and assessment that are coextensive to these. In addition, this antagonism partially defuses the popular and academic notions that depict a kind of conspiratorial ADHD connection between entities who are argued to effectively "fabricate" ADHD through their concerted action (Breggin 1998; Walker 1998). The interviews elucidate that although some clinicians may heavily rely upon the testimony of teachers, others want to maintain a degree of independence in determining whether or not a child with social/academic problems does in fact have a bona fide medical condition.

After Formal Assessments: Treating ADHD

At the conclusion of an ADHD assessment and probable diagnosis, it is important to analyze how treatment regimens are established by clinicians. As will be demonstrated, the application of different treatments speaks to the professional divisions that characterize the clinician sample. These divisions, such as those between pediatricians and clinical psychologists, are influential in the way clinicians perceive the nature of ADHD and frame ADHD children.

One of the primary factors that affect how a clinician will treat ADHD concerns the interpretation of a child's behavior. As a matter of course, this process of interpretation involves interaction among clinicians, parents, and teachers. As information is shared among these parties, certain treatment options become viewed as increasingly favorable. This type of interaction typifies the ADHD suspicion and diagnostic process, in which consultation among these adult figures formulates a profile of a suspected or diagnosed ADHD child. Consultations among adult authorities prior to the formal diagnosis and treatment of ADHD denotes that the framing of ADHD children is highly influential in how clinicians interpret their firsthand interactions with children and how clinicians link what they observe in these initial interactions to signs of ADHD. As information about a suspected ADHD child is sent down to a clinician's office, a "master frame" or overarching label (Carroll and Ratner 1996; Snow and Benford 1988) for an ADHD child is in its beginning stages of construction prior to initial visits to the clinic. As profiles of ADHD children are developed, both through interactions with such children and through discussions among adults, they become the foundation for a choice in treatment measures.

The celerity with which the master frame of an ADHD child is put forth strongly reflects which ADHD narrative (neurological, psychodynamic, or combination of the two) a particular clinician follows. When ADHD children are assessed comparatively fast—characterized by brief consultations with parents and teachers and by brief interactions with children in clinical settings, usually half an hour to an hour in length—the treatment is predominantly pharmacological. Furthermore, clinicians who perform relatively quick assessments of children are inclined to adopt a neurological perspective towards ADHD. Resonating well with the neurological perspectives explained in chapter 3, such clinicians view ADHD as a biochemical phenomenon, solved through medicinal means. In contrast, clinicians who take longer in applying a master frame to an ADHD child, or who never really subscribe to a consistent frame for such children, are more inclined to adopt a psychodynamic approach to the ADHD. The treatment methods such clinicians apply commonly involve behavior modification, psychotherapy, or related therapeutic means. Such clinicians are inclined to look at the learned nature of behavior and how the cultivation of metacognition and general self-awareness are integral to its treatment. Such clinicians are also more inclined to implicate family dynamics as a causal factor in the ADHD phenomenon and include family members in the therapy process. Non-psychiatric medical doctors seem the least inclined to adopt a psychodynamic approach to ADHD, except for those who are distinctly opposed to *DSM IV* criteria or see their diagnostic role as more than someone who applies a preordained label to children. Even those clinicians who subscribe to behavioral modification and family therapy do not always deny the usefulness of medications but instead emphasize the necessity to supplement pharmacological treatments with psychotherapy.

Bradley's Benzedrine

Prior to discussing clinicians' experiences in treating ADHD with medications, it is important to examine the history of stimulant medications and their relevance to how children with ADHD are perceived to be categorically different from other types of children.

The first account of children's reactions to stimulant medication is provided in Charles Bradley's (1937) article "The Behavior of Children Receiving Benzedrine."[1] Bradley commented that studies on adult responses to stimulant medications had been widely recognized but that nothing up to the time of his study had been published concerning the effect of stimulants on children.[2] His study sample consisted of thirty hospitalized children comprising a wide variety of mental disorder diagnoses:

> The children's behavior disorders were severe enough to have warranted hospitalization, but varied considerably. They ranged from specific educational disabilities, with secondarily disturbed school behavior, to the retiring schizoid child on the one hand and the aggressive egocentric epileptic child on the other (Bradley 1937, 578).

Bradley also mentioned that none of the children under study were mentally retarded, or markedly unintelligent: "The patients' intelligence was in general quite within the so-called 'normal range'" (Bradley 1937, 578). Despite this, all of these children, according to Bradley, were sufficiently mentally impaired to prevent them from functioning within conventional institutions. The children under study were institutionalized and out of mainstream life; however, the hospital within which they lived had periods of time throughout the day when conventional activities, such as schooling, occurred.

After the children had taken Benzedrine for only a few days, Bradley documented a dramatic alteration in the scholastic behavior of almost half of the study sample. One week after taking doses of Benzedrine, fourteen of the thirty children displayed "spectacular" improvement in school performance. With these fourteen children, "There appeared a definite 'drive' to accomplish as much as possible during the school period, and often to spend extra time completing additional work. Speed of comprehension and accuracy of performance were increased in most cases" (Bradley 1937, 578). Bradley also provided a detailed account of the children's emotional reaction to Benzedrine, which appeared to be "subdued," leading to overall improvements in social skills. These children, Bradley argued, demonstrated a greater interest in their surroundings and in other children. Bradley claimed that Benzedrine got children "out of themselves" and more constructively involved with their physical and social environment. He describes some of the children's comments:

> Although questioning the children in regard to their subjective feeling was studiously avoided in all instances, spontaneous remarks such as "I have joy in my stomach," "I feel fine and can't seem to do things fast enough today," "I feel peppy," "I start to make my bed and before I know it it is done" [were expressed by the children]. . . All of these patients showed a widening of interest in things around them, and superficially at least, a diminished tendency to be preoccupied with themselves (579).

Children's responses to the medication were not confined to performance in school. An improved performance and attitude were also visible in the ordinary events of daily life. Children on Benzedrine behaved in ways that mirrored some of the larger cultural expectations of what it means to be "well-adjusted." Self-centeredness—something Bradley saw as a common thread among all of these mentally disordered children, despite variation in diagnoses—was drastically reduced. Bradley's findings opened a new path in child neurology in which the effects of stimulants upon child behavior attained an immediate interest with his colleagues. Shortly after the publication of Bradley's seminal account, researchers would explore the relationship between Benzedrine and children's scores on intelligence tests (Motlitch and Eccles 1937), as well as the Stanford achievement test (Motlitch and Sullivan 1937).

Stimulant Medication and the Neurological Approach

In the forward to Paul Wender's *Minimal Brain Dysfunction in Children* (1971), Leon Eisenberg discusses the case history of a typical case of MBD, John, a seven-year-old who exhibited all the symptoms associated with the disorder. John's behavioral problems, which included severe hyperkinesis and impulsivity, are initially assessed by a psychotherapist and attributed to a family difficulty (Eisenberg in Wender, 1971, ix, x). Eisenberg claims that six months of psychotherapy in this case

> brought no obvious relief, and once the school insisted on re-
> tention in grade, the pediatrician sought help from consultation
> at a prominent medical center, where, at long last, the exis-
> tence of MBD was stated "authoritatively" on the basis of the
> total clinical picture. A trial of amphetamine therapy brought
> about striking behavioral changes, a decisive improvement in
> school performance, and a consequent uneasy peace among
> the "warring factions" (x).

For Eisenberg, this child's clinical profile reveals symptoms which are
not only associated with, but caused by, brain chemistry. John, in
Eisenberg's opinion, was someone with a clear-cut case of a physiological illness. The "warring factions" have no choice but to cease their conflict over the cause and cure of John's difficulties when amphetamine
therapy markedly reduces his symptoms. Eisenberg presents a case study
where the treatment of MBD with amphetamine is akin to providing an-
tibiotics for a bacterial infection. An organic cause requires a pharmacological cure. Eisenberg claims that the psychologists who initially assessed John

> had indeed noted real phenomena in this family; their error lay
> in ascribing causal priority to these issues because of a psy-
> chogenic bias whose origin is to be found in the one-sided na-
> ture of the clinical training of the orthopsychiatric team. The
> task of the medical center had been made easier by the interval
> history, but it was the response to stimulants that "settled" the
> dispute (x).

John's response to medications is seen as the great equalizer. The chemical interaction between medications and the brain, which can be seen in
visibly improved behavior, makes the case for a physiological understanding of MBD.

The clinicians I interviewed who were inclined to favor medication
(primarily pediatricians and general practitioners) as the sole method of
treatment for ADHD clearly sympathize with this neurological position.
This speaks again to the issue of what constitutes ADHD. From such clinicians' perspective, medication is appropriate for a legitimate neurological condition—what one respondent calls a "valid symptom category." Hence, clinicians who are highly favorable to medication therapy
for ADHD tend to claim that problem behaviors need to be addressed by

medications and that the many forms of psychotherapy largely are ineffective. Referring to a 1996 collaborative multimodal treatment assessment (MTA) study prompted in the United States by the National Institute of Mental Health, one general practitioner tells me, "The recent
MTA study clearly demonstrates that these work the best even when you
have someone doing both behavior modification and all of the other
kinds of therapies." This fourteen-month study measured the responses
of 579 ADHD children, ages seven through nine, to various treatment
methods, including behavior modification, combined treatment, and
medication treatment, and concluded that medication does more to cease
problem behaviors than any other approach to treating the disorder (see
Arnold 1997, Richters 1997, and Greenhill 1996 for discussions of this
study). The findings of this study have done much to bolster the opinions
of those who purport that ADHD is a truly neurological condition.

The results of the MTA study represent a continuation of the way the
diagnosis of ADHD has been validated in the research community.
Through arguing that medication is the most effective treatment for
ADHD, a neurological etiology of the disorder can be levied. In the tradi-
tion of Bradley's (1937) early stimulant studies, the MTA study further
solidifies a modality that argues that the nature of the ADHD ailment can
be understood through the child's response to medication—an act of reverse engineering that states the treatment defines the ailment it is treating. To be fair, it seems probable that Ritalin and other stimulants would
do the most to alter behavior, but would this not also be the case with
children who do not demonstrate ADHD symptoms?[3]

Enhancing Knowledge/Modifying Behavior

The subscription to non-pharmacological behavior modification reveals a
hesitation from some clinicians to embrace neurological maxims about
ADHD. Despite this, ADHD children who are perceived to need such
treatments are largely framed as "disabled." The belief in the effectiveness of behavior modification demonstrates that many clinicians seek the
remedy for ADHD-type behaviors through strategies for coping with different social contexts, rather than by simply administering medication.
Family units, for example, are routinely described as targets of ADHD
treatment. In mediating the treatment experience for families, many clinicians adopt the role of what I call "knowledge enhancers," claiming
that behavioral modification originates with the education of parents,

who need to have a thorough understanding of their child's condition in order for behavior modification to occur. As one clinician states: "We primarily try to educate parents and let them know a lot about their child's condition. ...We get parents into support groups, or we let them know where they are" (RN, manager of an ADHD clinic, age thirty-five). As "knowledge enhancers," clinicians appear wont to encourage parents to adopt a disability perspective, regardless of whether a child's ADHD is framed as psychodynamic or neurological. Such a perspective cultivates emotional detachment. Another clinician puts it this way: "Parents are usually very irritated and frustrated. Their kid is in all this trouble. ...Then we go over some techniques to help parents respond to their child, not react to what that child does" (clinical psychologist, age fifty-one).

Argued by psychodynamically oriented clinicians as a necessary step before the use of medication, behavior modification is repeatedly presented as a method for getting at the "root" of behavioral issues:

> Behavioral modification is the main thing I use. I like to see if they can get the kids off the meds before we start all of it. Then we can really know what some of the issues are, you know, behaviorally. I also counsel parents a lot, because when the kids are acting up there is usually something going on in the family. Martial issues are another big concern when I make assessments (clinical psychologist, age forty-seven).

The perception is that medication, in that it alters behavior, also obscures the environmental causes of these behaviors. Despite the prevalence of apparent neurological defect, many clinicians argue that ADHD has components that are rooted in other social environments. It is argued that a child struggling with difficulties in the home and then being prescribed medication for these problems has not adequately "dealt" with these issues. A child's cathartic emotional moments are argued to be obscured by medication.

Clinicians also state that parents need to develop self-regulatory mechanisms for how they will react to their children. In addition to developing a perspective that their child is disabled, parents are taught a certain degree of self-talk to keep them from provoking their children: "Working with parents on dealing with their child at home is probably the first thing we work on. ...I also try to teach parents coping statements like 'I can remain calm.' A lot of times parents blow up at their kids and with an ADDer that is not what you want to do. Things can really escalate" (clinical psychologist, age forty-two). ADHD children, therefore, are commonly regarded as volatile. The "ADDer" is clearly not a normal child in this sense. His/her volatility needs to be diluted through a carefully constructed interactive context whose boundaries are defined by the clinic and enforced in the domestic environment. One psychologist, for example, tells me the story of an eight-year-old ADHD child who was consistently late for school—his lateness being just one of his many ADHD symptoms. During a therapy session this child's mother was instructed by the psychologist to specify a time that the child was expected to be at the car and ready for school, "not *running* to the car at this time, but *at* the car at this time," the psychologist explains. The instructions were that if the child was not at the car at the specified time, the mother would drive off and leave him. The child's mother had an extremely difficult time with the enforcement of this rule, always fudging the time she allowed her son to get to the car. As the psychologist states: "the lateness problem did not go away." Finally, the day came when the mother drove off and left her son at home. This alteration in the mother's behavior is considered a behavior modification breakthrough by the psychologist: "He was rarely, if ever, late again," he states.

Behavior modification is also explained as a means to rectify the psychological problems specifically caused by medication, addressing, in this sense, both the condition of ADHD, and also the preeminent ADHD treatment: "If medication is prescribed by their doctor we will spend some time evaluating how the child is doing. Sometimes there can be some psychological problems associated with the medication and that needs to be dealt with immediately before anything else can really be effective" (clinical psychologist, age forty-five). The effect of medication, if not carefully evaluated, can be seen as a hindrance rather than a benefit to the behavior modification process. This reflects the sentiment of Lawrence Diller (1998), who argues that medication is a "necessary evil."

Uncertainty to Skepticism: Concerns about Prescribing Children Medication

Despite the fact that the "necessary evil" of medication is the most common treatment for ADHD in North America, there is considerable reservation about this treatment approach by clinicians in this sample. Numerous clinicians, for example, convey that Ritalin is probably overprescribed and that the ADHD diagnosis is given too freely. Other concerns that clinicians raise include risks of chemical dependency later in life, the removal of an internal locus of behavioral control, and the physiological side effects of medications. As I will demonstrate, many of these concerns resonate very strongly with discussions in popular and academic literature.

"Stimulant Medications Are Overprescribed"

The majority of reservations clinicians express about the use of stimulant medication primarily concern the inadequacy of the ADHD label. ADHD is perceived by many clinicians to have problems with its validity, including those described in chapter 3: the ambiguous language of *DSM IV*, the ADHD diagnosis failing to address more specific problems with an individual child, ADHD being a residual diagnosis, and so on. Such validity issues are something that have plagued the diagnosis of ADHD for over a century and contribute to the ongoing contested nature of the disorder. To date, there is no test that proves the existence of ADHD, and because the diagnosis cannot be conclusively validated, many clinicians argue that ADHD is diagnosed too frequently and with inadequate information. As one clinician states: "The diagnosis is given way too freely. That means more kids on meds who are not supposed to be on them or are too young for them. So, I think that if you're going to give meds, you should make sure you at least have the right diagnosis" (clinical psychologist, age forty-seven). And another clinician:

> I think ADHD is not a great diagnosis. It's an easy out for
> schools. They're under a lot of pressure, and they respond by
> trying to whip kids into shape. What about class size? What
> about more effective teaching strategies? I also think ADHD is
> a parenting issue a lot of times. Ritalin is the pacifier for kids,
> like TV and Nintendo (family therapist, age fifty-two).

Some clinicians view medications as a means to shirk fundamental issues underlying childhood behavioral problems: "It [medication] can be seen as a quick fix. Some people will go to a GP [general practitioner] or a pediatrician and get a quick and dirty diagnosis and a packet of pills, which is malpractice in my opinion. A pediatrician can easily just become a medication consultant, rather than someone who is really treating a real problem" (psychiatrist, age forty-seven). Some ADHD practitioners may feel others are too focused on the immediate behavior of the child they are treating. Rather than examining the greater social environment of that child, such clinicians may relegate themselves to the role of "medication consultants." Relieving the immediate situation of a child in crisis, some clinicians argue, is really to relinquish the responsibility to probe deeper into the child's circumstances.

The appropriateness of medication is also addressed by one respondent, who argues that its supposed effectiveness is akin to mythology:

> Well, the drug is simply inappropriate. It is a lie to think that any drug will make you smarter or better able to perform in school. If there was a drug to make you smarter I'd be taking it. But there isn't. Ritalin is a way of addressing the society's needs, but not the child's. With this little child's brain he needs blue and we give him red. Our society is not geared to children; it hates children, it sees them as a necessary nuisance. (points to sign on the wall that reads: "CHILDREN ARE NOT ADULTS.") That is why I have this up on the wall, to remind people that children are different (pediatrician, age forty-nine).

From this physician's perspective, Ritalin is a way to pacify the annoying behavior of children, rather than address the larger societal issues that make us so intolerant of them. His sign on the wall: CHILDREN ARE NOT ADULTS, is placed there as a reminder to parents that children behave differently from adults because *they are not* adults. Ritalin, from this perspective, makes children more somber, more adult-like, and is a way of "treating" childhood rather than a mental disorder. This respondent, a native of France, conveys that the intolerance of childhood behavior is uniquely North American. It was not until he moved from abroad that he saw apartment complexes where children were not allowed, or public displays of dislike for children's behavior. His account, while anecdotal, is not without merit. For example, citing a 1997 United Nations International Narcotics Control Board conference, PBS's *Frontline* reported that 90 percent of the world's Ritalin is consumed in the United States and Canada.

Concerns regarding the possible overprescription of Ritalin can be traced to broader concerns about the medical validity of ADHD and the conventional chemical methods with which it is treated. For example, in the fall of 1998, a National Institutes of Health conference of experts in ADHD research and treatment came to the unsettling conclusions that

ADHD, though an established part of the APA's nosology since 1987, has little consistency in diagnosis and may be treated capriciously (Goldman et al. 1998). This conference also addressed the fact that unlike other illnesses, there remains no test for ADHD that unequivocally confirms its existence. The results of PET scans, as reputable as they have been among North American researchers, are merely conjectural when postulating the biochemical nature of ADHD. There are a number of psychological instruments that measure rates of attention, concentration ability, and emotional responses to stressful situations, and these also have demonstrated scant reliability. Behavioral measurement instruments, such as the Conners Scale, SNAP IV, and Disruptive Behavior Disorder Scale, and attention measuring tests, such as the Continuous Task Performance Test, Wisconsin Card Sorting Test, Test of Variables of Attention, and Weschler Intelligence Scale for Children, are not adequate measuring devices for ADHD. Such scales may be adequate in providing accounts of how an individual responds to medication—and these tests are being increasingly used in that capacity—but they fail as a diagnostic measuring device (Goldman et al. 1998).

Furthermore, a Working Party of the British Psychological Association remains highly critical of the APA's description of ADHD, arguing that ADHD is a vacuous disease category (Reason 1999). This report also contends that the International Classification of Diseases (ICD) criteria for "hyperkinetic disorder" provides a much greater utility, as it is a set of criteria more stringent in its nosology, and would be more likely to reduce the alarmingly high prevalence of ADHD in North America. In light of such criticism of North American psychiatric practice and its conceptualization and treatment of ADHD, it would be premature to say that medication is the undisputed answer to ADHD.

Medication Psychoses

The uncertainty over whether or not medications are appropriate for unruly children is further demonstrated by clinicians who express concern about the drastic alterations in personality and possible psychotic reactions that can occur with the administration of such drugs. One clinician expresses these concerns and provides an example:

> I get really worried about side effects. It hasn't come up in a while, but some kids do not belong on meds. Some kids I've

> seen have developed other conditions. One kid became unusu-
> ally paranoid. He had some major unrealistic fears about other
> kids, about his siblings. We had to petition his parents and the
> doctor to get him off the drugs. The funny thing is his teachers
> felt like everything was fine. I tell you, he was not fine (clini-
> cal psychologist, age forty-five).

Another clinician provides this account: "A lot of the kids I've seen on meds are a lot more somber, not as happy. When the meds wear off, the kids can become over emotional, freak out, or get insomnia. You have to wonder how good the drug is working if that's what happens to the kids" (clinical psychologist, age fifty-six).

The concerns many clinicians express regarding the possible psychotic side effects of Ritalin and other drugs mirror numerous discussions in popular and academic literature. For example, in a brief article, "A Para-doxical Effect," Tracey Nicholls (1999) offers a biting commentary on the supposed and actual effects of stimulant medication. The "paradox" in the title of this article is that drugs, such as Ritalin, which are pur-ported in clinical circles to engender a reintegration into family and school activities and to increase chances of success for ADHD children, may actually cause antisocial, self-destructive behavior. Nicholls uses two provocative examples of known people who were prescribed Ritalin to back her claim, one being that of Nirvana front-man Kurt Cobain[4] who shot himself in 1994, the other, former Thurston High School student and mass murderer Kip Kinkel. In an argument as impassioned as it is non-scientific, Nicholls contends that Ritalin and drugs of its kind may foster feelings of hopelessness and outright psychosis.

Indeed, a great part of the historical record on stimulant drugs is lit-tered with discussions of their possible psychotic side-effects. The dis-cussion began in 1938, when two clinicians noticed psychotic symptoms in patients who were being treated with Benzedrine for narcolepsy (Young and Scoville 1938). The first of two cases these doctors describe is a thirty-four-year-old white male who, after being prescribed 20 to 30 mg. of Benzedrine a day, "became tense and anxious, feared for the safety of his family and had ideas of influence. He sought police protec-tion and believed his house was wired" (639). The second case involves a twenty-five-year-old white male the doctors describe as "exhilarated and self-conscious, thinking that people were noticing him and later that they were calling him a 'homo'" (640). Both of these cases, according to the authors, particularly displayed paranoid types of psychoses, feeling forces outside of their immediate control infiltrating their lives, plotting their demise, or attempting to stigmatize them. This paranoid component, according to the authors, may result from the increased sensitivity that ensues when Benzedrine is administered. They state: "The patient becomes more alert and observant; when extreme, this leads to ideas of reference and misinterpretation" (644).

With regard to adult patients, a plethora of literature addressing stimulant-based psychoses existed before the first prescriptions for Ritalin were written in 1961. This discussion culminated in what is arguably the most comprehensive treatment of the topic in P.H. Connell's *Amphetamine Psychosis* (1958). However, the first account of children's psychotic reactions to stimulants was not until Philip G. Ney's (1967) article "Psychosis in a Child Associated with Amphetamine Administration." This account begins with B.D., an eight-year-old boy who was receiving Dexedrine for "disruptive classroom behavior and poor performance at school. ...He was (also) fidgety, easily distractible, frustrated, disobedient, defiant and unable to follow directions" (1026). In addition, Ney contends that B.D. was "angry toward authority figures, but also had a great deal of self-blame for his failures" (1026).

Ney profiles B.D. as a patient in need of medical intervention and reports that the initial prescription for Dexedrine (5 mg, twice daily) showed results deemed favorable by those who subscribe to the gravity of the hyperkinetic syndrome. Behavioral improvements were apparently made both at school and at home after undergoing Dexedrine treatment, but these improvements gave way to unforeseen complications. As Ney describes:

> Suddenly one snowy day he appeared very perplexed and began talking about people throwing snowballs at him. Although he could not see these people, he could see the snowballs coming at him from behind and hitting him on the upper arm.
>
> On more detailed examination, he complained of people spying on him and talking about him although he could not figure out where the sound was coming from. ...He could not be persuaded that they [the hallucinations] were not real (1027).

As a result of this apparent state of psychosis, Ney withheld the medication to see if the hallucinations would disappear, which they did. However, after ceasing the medication, B.D.'s hyperkinetic symptoms returned, prompting Ney to place him back on Dexedrine albeit at an increased dosage (10 mg. in the morning, 5 mg. at noon). Ney describes the results: "With the increased dosage, he reported the telephone poles went 'blup blup' and on one occasion he jumped off the trampoline to look around the corner because he thought someone was there" (1027). Despite what appears to be a resurgence of B.D.'s psychosis, Ney dismisses this reaction, claiming it was less pronounced than those experiences B.D. previously described.

Ultimately, Ney concludes that B.D. may have had only a mild recurrence of psychosis and that these psychotic symptoms later disappeared. B.D., therefore, remained on the medication. Ney concludes his discussion: "It [this case of psychosis] poses many interesting theoretical questions and a practical dilemma. Since Bradley, in 1937, first reported the use of amphetamine in controlling hyperkinetic children,[5] it has been found that, although a paradoxical quieting may not always occur, when it does, it is quite dramatic" (1027). Ney relegates this case of child psychosis to the realm of "exception," rather than "rule." In that his response to Dexedrine was psychotic, rather than socially approved, the case of B.D. demonstrates an instance in which the "paradoxical quieting" did not result from Dexedrine administration. However, this instance is framed as an isolated occurrence and is not grounds for a larger critique of these medications.

The first report of child psychoses resulting from the administration of Ritalin was published in the *Journal of the American Medical Association* by Alexander Lucas and Morris Weiss in 1971. In this article, succinctly entitled "Methylphenidate Hallucinosis," the authors describe three cases: two girls, six-and-a-half and fifteen years of age, respectively, and one boy, age 10. All three children suffered from marked hallucinations. In the instance of the youngest girl, the authors report that

> her behavior became grossly bizarre. She cowered in a corner and hid in a closet. She had become apathetic and mute, failing to respond to her parents' questions. They stated that she appeared "almost like a vegetable." Occasionally, she shouted and struck out indiscriminately. She began to babble incoherently, stared into space glassy-eyed, and grimaced and contorted her body (1079).

The ten-year-old boy reported psychotic experiences that were more visual in nature. As the authors state: "When...questioned about his subjective experiences, he stated that he saw a rainbow and a whirlpool of colors. Lions, tigers, and elephants appeared to be marching around the whirlpool. He stated, 'I feel strong like I could tear everything apart'"

(1079-80). The oldest girl also described visual hallucinations: "Shadows in the woods seemed to materialize into people and bears. Objects such as logs were mistaken for animals" (1080).

For some researchers, the psychotic reactions that may accompany the use of stimulant medication are grounds for a complete reevaluation of such treatment methods. This "anti-Ritalin" discussion is most notably championed by Peter Breggin in *Talking Back to Ritalin* (1998), a text that is considered fundamental to today's criticism of the administration of stimulants to children. Breggin's work, perhaps more than any other, elaborates the "paradox" mentioned by Tracey Nicholls. In being one of the foremost critics of Ritalin use, Breggin represents considerable dissension within modern psychiatry and its discussion of stimulant medication. As a clinician, he provides an "insider's" perspective on the practice of prescribing Ritalin, and he devotes considerable space to the issue of psychosis. In describing such mental impairment, Breggin states:

> Toxic psychoses caused by stimulant drugs are usually different in important ways from what the lay person thinks of as being "crazy." Signs of general impairment in brain function are typically present, including confusion, memory loss, and perhaps disorientation. In medical terms, it can be called a delirium or acute organic brain syndrome to designate that overall brain function has been impaired. Hallucinations, if they occur, are commonly visual and may involve seeing and feeling small creatures, like bugs. The experience is usually terrifying (16).

Breggin continues to say that such psychoses in children usually end when stimulant medication is ceased. However, he also mentions the residual effects of such psychotic episodes, describing their possible lasting impact upon a child:

> Even if full recovery seems to occur, the individual may be left with a variety of fears and anxieties. I have evaluated patients who were considered fully recovered by previous physicians but who continue to display residual effects, including recurrent strange ideas or sensations, insecurity, and fearfulness (16).

This passage represents a perspective on children that defies some of the mechanical perspectives taken by neurology, namely, that childhood misbehavior results from a physical process with discernible mechanisms and remedies. In describing the possibility that the immediate effects of psychoses may give way to longer lasting residual ones, Breggin humanistically asserts that children and their mental aberrations cannot be turned on and off like a switch.

Removing the "Internal Locus of Control" through Cosmetic Psychopharmacology

In addition to concerns about the physical side-effects of Ritalin and other drugs were concerns about such drugs' impact on the social psychological relations of a child. Some clinicians explain that children's identity as understood by both themselves and the adult authorities in their lives, often became dependent on the continued use of medication. The "locus of control" of the child, as one respondent put it, is placed upon an outside, chemical medium, rather than on the development of the child's own social and academic skills: "And then there's the issue of parental responsibility. Mothers will often say: 'He's acting like that because he didn't take his medication today.' There's no internal locus of control. It's all about the meds" (clinical psychologist, age forty-two). In order to evaluate the level of loss of the internal locus of control, it is argued that children need to be evaluated in order to demonstrate the extent that improved behavior remained after ceasing medication:

> One thing that is concerning me more and more is the dependency upon the medication for continued good behavior. I sometimes see children who I feel should stop taking the medication or should attempt it anyway, and they sort of refuse that. It's like the child cannot be a good boy unless the medication is around. ...There needs to be more independence from the effects the drug has upon behavior, allow people to kind of stand on their own and see how they do without it (pediatrician, age forty-three).

Parents and other authority figures, this response illustrates, are resistant to the idea of ceasing medication because it is believed to be the primary linchpin between the child and appropriate conduct.

This issue mirrors those mentioned in Peter Kramer's well-known, *Listening to Prozac* (1993). In the first chapter, "Makeover," Kramer describes the case of a female patient suffering from depression whose identity becomes transformed by this new drug called Prozac. Through its use, she experiences rapid and remarkable personal improvements, and becomes admittedly dependent upon the drug for her new identity, dubbing herself "Ms. Prozac" (12). When the marked improvement in her life becomes grounds for her to be taken off the drug, the patient states that she did not "feel like herself." As Kramer says: "This is not a question of addiction or hedonism, at least not in the ordinary sense of those words, but of having located a self that feels true, normal, and whole, and of understanding medication to be an occasionally necessary adjunct to the maintenance of that self" (20). Kramer eventually places her back on Prozac, rhetorically asking the reader: "Who was I to withhold from her the bounties of science?" (10).

Kramer expresses concern about the return of clinical depression when many of his patients are taken off Prozac and ponders whether or not dependencies on this drug are more for personality enhancements than for medical issues. He ultimately concedes to the benefits of Prozac, giving in to the new era of what he calls "cosmetic psychopharmacology" (15). Within this new realm of psychiatric practice clinicians are presented with the dilemma of prescribing medications not just for specified mental affectations but for flaws in character or simply to improve one's performance in certain social contexts. Clinicians who have concerns about patients' dependency upon Ritalin for continued good behavior, yet continue to prescribe the drug, are caught up in this same dilemma. The correction of behavior and the relief of immediate crises take precedence over addressing the way the ADHD child's self-concept becomes intertwined with stimulant medication.

Stimulant Medication and Concern about Chemical Dependency

Among other concerns clinicians express about stimulant use is the possibility that a prescription for Ritalin will lead to drug abuse later in the child's life. As one clinician states: "I am really afraid of issues of chemical dependency. I don't think that Ritalin is that much different from something like meth, and if you're taking that drug every day, it seems like it will lead to some severe problems" (psycho-educational assessor, age thirty-six). Another respondent contends that the use of Ritalin could be dangerous in a family that may already have a tendency towards drug abuse: "It seems like a lot of the kids I see already have a familial propensity for drug abuse, and Ritalin may make that worse" (child psychologist, age fifty-five). This concern over Ritalin being a precursor to illicit substance abuse later in life is very similar to the issues of Ritalin and the locus of control in the ADHD child. We may ask whether or not the dependency on Ritalin for improved behavior motivates the child taking the drug to be more inclined to view other drugs positively, but how warranted this inquiry would be remains to be seen. A 1999 University of California at Berkeley study argued that childhood use of Ritalin increases the possibility of using other substances, such as cigarettes, alcohol, and cocaine. However, this study was later refuted by a Massachusetts General Hospital study that concluded providing Ritalin to ADHD kids actually prevented later drug abuse (Chase 1999).

Despite the lack of consensus on whether Ritalin is a factor in later drug abuse, or is itself an abuse hazard, writers continue to frame Ritalin unfavorably. For example, in a recent *Christian Science Monitor* article, Alexandra Marks (2000) argues that Ritalin abuse is an increasing concern in North America: "In public schools and private universities across North America, Ritalin is increasingly the drug of choice for thousands of young people, from 10-year-old grade-schoolers dabbling with a first illicit high to graduate students in need of an all night push to finish a term paper" (1). In addition, an article in the *Chronicle of Higher Education* states that Ritalin, in conjunction with other drugs, such as heroin and alcohol has become a legitimate health hazard for college students (Nicklin 2000). The underlying argument in such articles is that Ritalin is a "gateway drug" whose use in grammar and high school eventually opens the door to full-fledged drug abuse.

When to Stop the Meds

As with other mood altering medications, stimulants have a tremendous variability in how they are prescribed. This includes constraints about what times these drugs are taken, in what dosages, who dispenses the medication, and so forth. Of particular interest here are the conditions under which clinicians feel that ADHD children could temporarily cease taking medication, what one respondent refers to as a "medication holiday."

The "Medication Holiday"

Because ADHD behaviors are most commonly suspected in the school context, medication is often prescribed as a response to the demands of that environment. Therefore, the majority of clinicians state that when the demands of school are not present, the medication becomes less necessary. This includes weekends, Christmas vacations, summertime, and so on:

> We do recommend that parents take their kids off the meds when the environment isn't as demanding. Holidays are always a good time to get off the meds and allow the body to readjust. Sometimes that doesn't work very well—parents say 'get him back on!'—but sometimes it's really necessary. (clinical psychologist, age forty-five).

And another clinician:

> During summertime they should take breaks and wash 'em out a little bit. I'm often curious to know what kind of learning explorations they do during those breaks. I think that seeing how kids behave without structure can help us see what kind of learners they are (clinical psychologist, age thirty-nine).

Because it requires behavior ADHD kids are supposedly unable to demonstrate, the "demanding" environment of school is contrasted with the less demanding, less structured circumstances of summer break. The term "summer" describes a block of time during a calendar year, certainly, but it is also a euphemism for being "outside of school." During this period of time, clinicians say that a child may be allowed to engage in explorations that are not mediated by medication. The ADHD child, from this perspective, can be better understood through his/her experiences in an unregulated, unmedicated environment. By stating that children without structure can reveal their inherent learning strategies, this excerpt partially disputes the idea that treating ADHD may render "normal" the condition in the child's brain. Normalcy is relative in this instance, the child being framed as merely a different type of learner rather than truly pathological. This diverts attention from the child's pathology toward the school, which may be viewed in this instance as too demanding, too structured, etc. While within the learning environment of school, the ADHD child's nature impedes success, but when the child is removed from those rigid confines, this impediment seemingly disappears.

There is also a physiological concern that is common with respondents who incorporate taking breaks from medication into their treatment protocol. Many implied that the medication, even though it may be fixing problem behaviors and is beneficial in one sense, is undeniably a foreign element in the body. As one respondent states: "We can't constantly remain on a drug. Our bodies will start to break down" (clinical psychologist, age forty-five). Another clinician, whose son is diagnosed with ADHD, is more blunt about her opinion on the cessation of medication:

> I am supposed to say that that is a medical issue, but kids are
> on it too bloody long. I used to have my kid's teacher make
> him run laps when he acted out. He was never medicated and
> he really got into shape from all of the running. We still joke
> about that (clinical psychologist, age fifty-six).

With rare exception, the clinicians I spoke with acknowledge that Ritalin alters bodily chemistry in an unnatural way. Another respondent discusses the side effects of Ritalin, primarily its ability to reduce caloric intake:

> I will recommend a break from the meds if there is a consis-
> tent lack of caloric intake. That is one of the common side ef-
> fects, lack of appetite. With the younger ones we have to
> really watch that. We give them a break so they can eat nor-
> mally and get their calorie count on par with others their age
> (pediatrician, age forty-seven).

The theme of the "medication holiday" reflects some of the perceived purposes of medication. We may ask: Is medication more than a means to better school behavior? Is medication also a learning device that enables ADHD children to develop social as well as academic skills? From the vast majority of respondents, the answer is no. Ritalin is seen as necessary to settle down disruptive behavior and to facilitate the mechanics of learning, but is not argued to be entirely necessary in other environments.

Notes

1. To examine later researcher accounts of stimulant medications and children, please see Conners and Eisenberg (1963); Douglas et al. (1969); Eisenberg et al. (1963); and Eisenberg (1972).

2. Charles Bradley is considered to be the most significant contributor to the early study of children and stimulant medications, not just due to his 1937 account, but also due to his other publications that postulated stimulant drugs to be a viable treatment for childhood behavioral problems. For example, see Bradley and Bowen (1940), Bradley and Green (1940), and Bradley and Bowen (1941). It was also Bradley (1950) who first claimed that Dexedrine may be superior to Benzedrine for treating problem children.

3. I am reminded of recreational Ritalin users who use this stimulant in the same capacity they would marijuana or methamphetamine. The recreational user of Ritalin certainly uses the drug for effect—something that would clearly be demonstrable through changes in behavior. The case of the recreational user of Ritalin is grounds for arguing that Ritalin is not only effective in children with ADHD. That being said, it could also be retorted that recreational users of Ritalin are *really* ADHD to some capacity and are using Ritalin and other drugs as a way of "self-medicating."

4. In *the Hyperactivity Hoax* (1998), Sydney Walker also mentions Kurt Cobain as an example of the psychological damage Ritalin may cause.

5. This assertion is inaccurate. Bradley's (1937) account mentions institutionalized children with a variety of apparent mental illness problems, and never invokes the phrase "hyperkinetic syndrome"—a nomenclature which would not become used in clinical circles for another thirty years.

Chapter Five

The Realm of Semiformal Suspicion:
Framing ADHD in the Classroom

In contrast to clinicians, who experience ADHD cases in a rather exclusive diagnostic and treatment capacity, teachers' roles with respect to ADHD children are multifaceted. Teachers are influenced by their own acceptance, or lack thereof, of the validity of ADHD, by how they see ADHD children as differing from others, and by the extent to which they have knowledge of ADHD and apply these understandings to the children they suspect of having the disorder. Highlighted by the accounts previously given from clinicians, the present chapter will elaborate how teachers are integral social actors in beginning the social organizational response to a perceived act of deviance. For the purposes of sociological investigation, the extent to which teachers suspect children of having ADHD and draw more formalized attention to these suspicions is of great importance. The ways in which teachers suspect children of having ADHD and consequently approach outside parties with these suspicions demonstrates the influx of clinical ADHD knowledge into the classroom environment and into the professional domain of teachers.

ADHD and the Classroom

As chapter 4 demonstrates, ADHD is associated more with schools than with any other institutional context. This can be seen in the way pharmacological treatments for ADHD have been and continue to be justified, and also in how the current APA criteria for ADHD directly implicate the school environment. Past and present advertisements in medical and psychiatric journals for drugs such as Ritalin and Cylert commonly employ scholastic themes, and *DSM IV* criteria for ADHD appear to have been written largely with classroom situations in mind. This linkage between ADHD and the specific context of schools demonstrates the influence of past ADHD discourse. Of particular interest here is the early discussion of how ADHD symptoms were deemed pathological because they apparently prevented children from learning school lessons. This type of conceptualization of ADHD symptoms can be found in both the discussion of the 1920s psychiatric sequelae of *encephalitis lethargica* and the later psychodynamic perspectives on the disorder that explained overt behavioral problems as resulting from frustrations with institutional environment, the school being primary in this regard.

The association between ADHD suspicion and the classroom is drawn from those on both the pro and con side of the ADHD debate. Those skeptical of the validity of ADHD label the school as an institution where antagonism between staff and student is rectified through mental disorder labels. (For a scathing critique of the school system's role in identifying hyperactivity see Shrag and Divoky [1975]). On the other hand, those who subscribe to the validity of ADHD will identify the school as a crucial context for discovering this potentially devastating disorder. For example, in *Children on Medication* (1986) Kenneth Gadow summarizes the role of the school system in the life of an ADHD-diagnosed child: "The school is often in the middle of this controversy because it is: a) frequently the source of medical referral, b) intimately involved in fostering academic achievement, and c) one of the most challenging settings for the hyperactive child" (31-32). Gadow portrays the school as a major catalyst to ADHD diagnoses. Due to the particular intellectual and social demands it places upon children, Gadow argues that the school is where the signs of ADHD are most visible, and, because schools are perceived to be crucial in improving one's future quality of life, to not recognize children who may have ADHD is to abandon them to a host of social ills.

Education literature demonstrates a growing interest in those who have or are suspected of having ADHD. An examination of a cross-section of this literature reveals the extent to which the discussion of ADHD has become commonplace in teaching circles (Bloomingdale 1985; McCall 1989; Buchoff 1990; Black 1992). Take, for example, an article in *Instructor* magazine, "How To Manage Your Students with ADD/ADHD" adapted from Linda J. Pfiffner's *All about ADHD* (1996):

> Odds are you have one or two students in your classroom who have ADD or ADHD—attention deficit (hyperactivity) disorder. As you know well, these students are not easy to teach. Their high rate of movement and talkativeness may be difficult to handle.
> . . . ADD students are challenging even for the most seasoned teachers. Getting them to focus, pay attention, and follow directions can be like trying to herd cats (63).

The article then describes a variety of methods that can be employed to effectively teach ADHD children, including classroom layout and student-teacher interaction models that minimize distractions, and rigid lesson plans that provide extra structure. Similar articles emphasize the necessity of providing outlets for ADHD children, for example, using an "acting out" room for times when the impulse to misbehave is greater than the child's own willpower (Dyer-Wiley 1999).

In addition to addressing techniques on how to cope with ADHD children, numerous studies also argue for teachers to become effective ADHD diagnosticians. Recent articles in journals such as the *School Psychology Review* and *Teacher Education and Special Education* repeatedly stress the importance of teachers playing both an intervention role with regard to ADHD children and an intermediary role between the child's domestic and clinical environments (Greene 1995; Power and DuPaul 1996; Sheridan et al. 1996; Schultz et al. 1997). In order to mold teachers into these roles, such studies claim that extensive knowledge of ADHD is imperative. An article by McFarland, Kolstad, and Briggs (1995) exemplifies this urgency. In a section subtitled "The Teacher's Role in Diagnosing and Teaching ADHD Children," the authors provide a case for the inevitability of an educator's encountering an ADHD child and an admonishment for teachers to learn to recognize such a child:

> Educators play an important role in diagnosing and treating ADHD children...Teachers must have an awareness of ADHD symptoms and the methods of treating this abnormality.
>
> Although virtually all elementary classroom teachers would prefer to go through their careers without encountering an ADHD student, this very likely will not be the case.
>
> ...What should teachers do to prepare for this inevitable encounter with an ADHD student? The first thing teachers must do is to develop an understanding of ADHD behavior so they can help in the diagnosis of the condition. The teacher's training programs should include sufficient information to help identify possible cases of ADHD (601).

The increasing recognition of ADHD in the classroom has also been used to examine the clinical criteria for ADHD. One study, for example, utilizes questionnaire data provided by school teachers to evaluate the validity of *DSM IV*'s criteria for ADHD and concludes that the understanding of ADHD within the educational environment represents a parallel understanding to that of the American Psychiatric Association

(Wolraich 1996). Such studies clearly demonstrate a point of interaction between formal medical nomenclature and the production of ADHD knowledge in the classroom setting. It may be argued that with regard to ADHD and perhaps other childhood mental disorders, there is an inter-dependent relationship between educational and medical knowledge, in which the everyday experience of educators is used as validation for the postulates generated in the medical realm. Illuminating the connection between medicine and education are the ways in which the teachers I interviewed conceptualize ADHD children and use such conceptual frameworks to separate them from the general student population.

Distinguishing ADHD Students from "Normal" Students

In framing ADHD students, teachers universally articulate that there are drastic and discernible differences between children with the disorder and normal children. The perception of these differences formulates how children who are perceived to be "in trouble" could be teased out of the regular student population and given what teachers would argue to be appropriate accommodation. Teachers' conceptions of ADHD children reflect a belief in fundamental differences between children achieving academic and/or social success in the classroom and those who struggle in these areas. By using the word "fundamental," I mean that teachers by and large saw ADHD as an impassable impediment to participation in the social and academic exchanges in school. Teachers tend to extrapolate that these basic problems affect all areas of a child's life. The manner in which they distinguish ADHD children implicates both academic and social problems. That is, teachers argue that ADHD can be seen in some children's difficulty in meeting the challenge of work-related tasks, and also in their difficulties with other students. With regard to school work, ADHD children are often described as having less of an ability to maintain focus and stay on task than their non-ADHD peers. With regard to social situations, ADHD children are described as antagonistic toward others, due in part to what some teachers claim is an inability to pick up on the types of social cuing other students respond to automatically.

"They Can't Stay on Task"

Coinciding with the descriptions of ADHD in *DSM IV*, teachers consistently frame ADHD children as unable to maintain focus and complete given tasks. Of most concern is that this lack of focus affects academic performance. As one teacher states: "It's hard for them to maintain focus, to maintain any kind of focus. They have bad follow through, bad organization skills. It's really hard for them to follow any kind of lengthy direction" (seventh grade teacher, age forty-four). And another teacher: "Well, in their hyperactivity, their inability to concentrate. Some may have really erratic impulses, you know, do things which are way out of line. ...But, the concentration and focus, that's a big one" (sixth grade teacher, age fifty-five). ADHD children, it is argued, have a block that prevents the completion of significant school-related tasks. Teachers contend that such children's impulsivity may lead them to approach a topic or assignment with enthusiasm, but because they lack the ability to follow through on what they begin, their scholastic careers are littered with incomplete projects. For many teachers, this is a curious and frustrating aspect of the ADHD condition: ADHD children, many teachers contend, are prone to explore new ideas, and had in fact a tenacious enthusiasm for many topics; however, when it came time for the realization of these ideas, they had already moved on to something more interesting. In addressing these concerns, some teachers speak to the conflict between the personality of ADHD children and school curricula: "It's almost like we are dealing with different types of learners altogether with these kids. Maybe some kids just need to 'spaz' out in all kinds of directions before they find something that really grabs them. ...I guess the problem is that most schools don't work that way" (third grade teacher, age thirty-four).

Further expressing the frustration that some teachers feel with ADHD children is the idea that such children have potential to be high achievers if they could just be properly aided in focusing on important tasks. As one teacher states: "Well, I think these kids are very bright and intelligent but don't get things done the way they are supposed to. ...They have this tremendous imagination, but they can't seem to pull it all together" (fourth, fifth, and sixth grade teacher, age forty-two). ADHD children's higher level of activity, in this regard, can be attributable to having high intelligence and imagination. Another respondent also describes ADHD children as having a more active intellect than other children:

> I think they have a more active mind. They're very easily
> stimulated by things outside of what is supposed to be the fo-
> cal point. They need a tremendously intense experience to fo-
> cus adequately. Like when you put them in front of a com-
> puter, you can keep their attention (fourth grade teacher, age
> fifty-one).

The ADHD child's intellect is explained as more demanding, requiring a concentrated dose of stimulation in order to become focused. This same teacher reflects this perspective on ADHD through a story of a fourth grade ADHD boy who had intense classroom problems and found himself in the principal's office on numerous occasions. Upon one visit to the principal, the boy, while in the waiting area of the main office, noticed that the secretary was having some trouble with her computer. Her colleagues were standing over her shoulder trying to troubleshoot the problem, but to no avail. After watching this for a while, the boy told them that he knew the solution to the computer problem. Giving up on their own resources, the secretary and surrounding troubleshooters allowed the boy to have a go at it. Within a few minutes the boy fixed the computer problem and effectively explained how to avoid it in the future. Since that time, the staff at his school has asked him, on more than a few occasions, to assist in the repair of computer difficulties. As his teacher explains, "This was a kid flunking out of school, but who had spent hours in front of a computer." In a reversal of the clinical stereotype of ADHD children as neurologically underactivated and disabled, such a story casts these children in a much more favorable, and socially acceptable, light. ADHD may even be seen as a gift through such narrative.

Other teachers elaborate on the discussion of the inability to concentrate on conventional classroom projects as an example of a different learning propensity: "They have difficulty attending to one task and a real difficulty with seat work. They're much better at hands on work" (seventh grade teacher, age thirty-eight). Such a perspective denotes ADHD children as having the possibility for more academic success if provided the means to achieve it. This excerpt also describes ADHD children as more of what many teachers call a "kinesthetic learner," or those who learn through the physical manipulation of objects. Underlying this notion is that ADHD children have difficulty conceptualizing without the use of the hands. Their learning is articulated as a more physical process, and indeed, "ADHD learners" are repeatedly described in the interviews as more physically oriented than their non-ADHD peers.

The narrative of the ADHD learner is also implicit in responses that depict ADHD children as processing information differently. As one teacher states, ADHD children differ

> in the ways they process information and react to stimuli. They process more kinds of information at once and can't really sort out the different messages that are being transmitted to them. I think their reactions to things also vary. They may be overwhelmed by something another kid just shrugs off. It's like they're sensitive to things in odd ways (seventh grade teacher, age forty).

ADHD children are framed as having an inability to sort out the stream of different stimuli that comes at them in a classroom environment—a contention that clearly maintains such children are wired differently. Furthermore, behavioral difficulties are explained as a result of frustration with the child's inability to adequately function in the classroom environment. This position resonates with psychodynamic stances taken toward ADHD symptoms, namely, that ADHD-related behavior may be the result of not being able to make sense of a bombardment of information. Such children, the reasoning goes, reach a point of being "overwhelmed" and are compelled to act out.

ADHD Children as "Socially Disabled"

Based upon assumptions about ADHD children's inability to comprehend information, Dale R. Jordan (1988) emphasizes ADHD children's lack of self-awareness and their tendency to have slower social development:

> The ADD syndrome child seldom comprehends more than 30% of what occurs around him or her. ...New vocabulary is not added to the language stock on schedule. New data is not fully recorded by the mind. There is no steady, ongoing growth of skills in academic work or social development (29).

The skills that other children develop, including social skills, are missed by this type of child. ADHD children, in Jordan's opinion, are socially maladjusted. They have the ability to formulate some types of relationships and feel emotions but ultimately cannot express these appropriately. Jordan states: "Most ADD syndrome youngsters are likable in one-to-one relationships. ...These children are often deeply sensitive, feeling the same emotions felt by other sensitive youngsters. They care deeply for pets" (29). The pet-loving ADHD children are depicted as having the emotional qualities of "normal" social actors yet not having the neurological prowess to express these and involve themselves in a reciprocating relationship with their social environment. They are inclined to become socially isolated.

Such isolation can lead to a litany of disciplinary problems, which, as psychologists stated decades earlier, are due to the frustration incurred from consistent failure, especially within school: "These children bring a cluster of problems into the classroom" (Jordan 1988, 29). A consistent frustration with the outside world fuels a growing self-centeredness in ADHD children. They fail to recognize the effects their actions have upon others. In Jordan's (1988) words:

> Inattention makes it impossible for the ADD syndrome child to recognize the need to put self aside in the interest of others. ...Hyperactive ADD syndrome children act out their inner stories, rocking their chairs, turning furniture upside down for fortresses (30).

Teachers I interviewed also argue that a primary difference between ADHD children and their non-ADHD peers could be seen in the former's exhibition of disruptive behavior. As one teacher states: "With the kids who are unmedicated, their behavior is a lot worse. I've had kids doing all kinds of things in here, you know, hiding under the table, barking like a dog" (special education teacher, age forty-five). And another teacher: "They get just plain crazy, but you take a step back and you can see something is wrong there. They don't realize what they're doing" (second grade teacher, age forty-two). This lack of awareness, some teachers argue, translates into interpersonal problems. In contrast to the positions of Dale Jordan (1988), depicting ADHD children as having success in more intimate, one-on-one settings, such teachers are inclined to describe ADHD children as having an all-encompassing social ineptness. As one teacher states: "They also have a really hard time creating deeper relationships with other kids. As they get older, that becomes really apparent. When they're younger it's not as obvious. It's like the class clown starts becoming more of a serious social problem" (sixth and seventh grade teacher, age thirty-four). The "class clown," regarded as funny by children and a tolerable nuisance by teachers, becomes viewed as truly maladjusted as he/she gets older. For many teachers, ADHD children's neurological defects are perceived integral to why they repeatedly had difficulties with other children. As one teacher states: "They don't understand the idea of a boundary or a limit" (third and fourth grade teacher, age forty-seven). Such boundaries and limits include the social interaction rules that are an established part of public school curricula and also the personal boundaries of other students. As they are reputed to lack awareness of the demarcated boundaries of conduct, children with ADHD are portrayed as socially disabled.

These social disabilities, teachers argue, translate into directly confrontational behavior. One respondent states that "they are so impetuous...getting into fights on the playground. I'd say half the time when a fight occurs it's usually involving one of the ADD kids" (sixth grade teacher, age fifty-five). Others emphasize that even though ADHD kids are often involved in physical disputes at school, they are not always the aggressor in such altercations:

> I think they do get into fights more than the non-ADHD kids, but I don't think they're always the ones starting it. Some of these kids have a target painted right on their forehead and the other kids just go for it. They really take aim on them (special education teacher, age forty-four).

ADHD children's tendency to fight is not always a result of neurological dysfunction but results from the way other kids respond to their disabilities. In stating that "some of these kids have a target painted on their forehead," this teacher conveys the social vulnerability of ADHD children. Academic shortcomings, failure to formulate strong social bonds, and other social and psychological manifestations of ADHD are argued to be weakness areas that other children exploit. Furthermore, in instances in which they are the alleged aggressors, ADHD children are commonly portrayed as responding to cruelty they could no longer tolerate. In discussing the involvement of ADHD children with violence—either as victim or perpetrator—the explanations vary, but generally adhere to psychodynamic explanations. ADHD children, in this capacity, are described as frustrated not only by the mental demands of the learning environment but also by its social demands. In social situations there is a notion that individuals should maintain a certain thickness of skin, a certain tolerance to the prodding of others. For ADHD children, who are clearly framed as lacking some of these tolerance thresholds, it may be argued that withstanding the teasing assault of other kids is impossible.

In accordance with the themes of volatility that characterize the discourse of ADHD, teachers also express that failing to treat ADHD was to risk having to later reckon with an ADHD child's propensity for violence. In one instance, this perspective equated ADHD children's volatility with that of other neurologically disabled kids. As one teacher states: "Much like the FAS (fetal alcohol syndrome) kids, the ADHD kids just kind of placidly go with the flow and then they finally explode. There's a real potential for violence in some of them" (sixth grade teacher, age fifty-five). This potential for violence is also linked to ADHD children as having a different thought process and a different perception of what constituted a threat:

> I think you have to understand that ADHD kids aren't thinking the same as other kids. They may see something as threatening that you or I don't. If you act wrongly towards them, they may lash out at you. They might do some real damage too. So, if we can intervene and get them thinking on the right track they become normal, like other kids (second and third grade teacher, age forty-seven).

Treatment of the ADHD condition is argued in this passage to be an important part of putting such children's thinking back in line with conventional standards. If effectively addressed, the thought process of ADHD children can be augmented to reduce their volatility.

In connection with their diminished capacity for understanding social situations, ADHD children are commonly described by most teachers as incorrigible if they are not treated through medical channels. Disciplinary mechanisms as simple as telling a student to stay seated are articulated as fruitless in dealing with untreated ADHD children. As one teacher puts it: "The ones I've had, you tell them to sit down and they're right back up again. Two minutes later or three minutes later they're back at it again, over and over. You know as a teacher that they completely forgot what you just told them" (seventh grade teacher, age forty). According to many teachers, the repeated failure of conventional remedial action in the classroom is the basis for formal intervention: "At some point you have to say, 'OK, the kid's not learning anything here.' Then its time to consider some of the other options" (second grade teacher, age forty-two). These additional options include having such children psychiatrically evaluated.

ADHD as a "Non-Human Agent"

In providing reasons for why ADHD children act out, teachers rarely point to a student's own willful neglect of commonly understood school rules or social boundaries. Nor did teachers give any significant attention to family problems as a possible factor in an ADHD child's difficulties. The ADHD condition is repeatedly articulated as an entity that supplants the better intentions of such children. ADHD is cast as a "non-human agent" (Weinberg 1997) that compels certain types of behavior and when applied to ADHD represents an interesting marriage between psycho-dynamic and neurological perspectives on the disorder. Resonating with a psychodynamic view of ADHD, the frustrations children experience when failing in the school environment supersede their own desires for social acceptance and the avoidance of trouble. According to teachers' interpretations of events in their classrooms, frustrations get the better of ADHD kids, and they invariably act inappropriately. From a neurological perspective, we see consistent allusion to physical disabilities. Teachers appear firmly engrossed in the idea that ADHD students have a brain that processes information poorly. Hence, their learning and behavioral diffi-culties do not stem from family problems, struggles with particular stu-dents, or inept teaching, but are from a somatic source.

The apparently constant conflict that ADHD children have with school leads many teachers to argue that the disorder, if left untreated, is impos-sible to control: "I really don't know if they can adequately control them-selves once they get the urge to do something. So, when they get in trou-ble we act like they are supposed to understand how to control them-selves? ...someone has to intervene here, you know, do something that we (referring to teachers) really aren't equipped to do" (special education teacher, age forty-four). From this perspective, teachers must appropri-ately understand that the actions of ADHD children stem from something that the children themselves cannot control. Children, the reasoning con-tinues, do not have a desire to get into trouble, and the ones who find themselves always in the principal's office could not realistically want this type of social isolation. Hence, statements such as "we act like they are supposed to understand how to control themselves," elucidate the futility of conventional interpretations of ADHD behavior, reemphasiz-ing the disability perspective and non-human agency.

In that it places blame for disruptive behavior upon a non-human agent, the disability perspective invariably favors non-human forms of intervention, namely, medication. As one teacher states:

> For a teacher to say "pay attention" is not always effective. It's a stimuli issue, more than a disciplinary one. I'm not a huge fan of medication, but it works, in a miraculous way, sometimes. Yeah, they definitely need help. They want to pay attention, but the impulse is beyond them (special education teacher, age forty-five).

Conventional perspectives on classroom misbehavior are perceived to be ineffective with ADHD children. As this teacher proclaims, ADHD is not an issue about discipline but is rather an issue about the way ADHD children process the world. The impulse these children receive to behave in a particular way is beyond the scope of their own self-control. Because of this condition, medication is seen as a necessary intervention strategy. Such sentiments overwhelmingly represent the collective opinion of the teachers I interviewed. Though not all teachers I interviewed favored medication, most feel that it is necessary to curtail severe behavioral problems.

It is important to mention, however, that a minority of the teachers I interviewed adopt a developmental, rather than a disability, stance toward ADHD, arguing that the disorder may become less severe as a child matures or successfully deals with difficult things in life: "Kids need time sometimes to sort out their own stuff, their own life problems. I guess with all the demands it's not that easy for them, but sometimes I really feel that a lot of these kids grow out of their problems" (third grade teacher, age thirty-six). Another respondent, who is skeptical of the use-value of medication, emphasizes maturity as a major factor in the cessation of ADHD behavior:

> Some kids just outgrow it. As they mature, things become more calm, mellowed out. That's why meds are something I'm not too sure about. If the kid is going through a phase of his emotional development, is it a good idea to medicate when the phase becomes difficult for people? (fifth, sixth and seventh grade teacher, age forty).

The burden of responsibility, in this regard, is placed upon adults surrounding troubled children who may not have a bona fide mental disorder but may be struggling with a normal phase of living. This passage implies that the wrong type of intervention on behalf of intolerant and/or impatient adults may effectively cheat a child out of the possibility of attaining social and emotional maturity.

The Gentle Way in Diagnosing

Now that we have explored some of the major ways in which ADHD children are framed by teachers, it is important to analyze the methods and resources they use in beginning formal interventions with such children. Through analyzing the ways and means by which teachers draw formal attention to ADHD-suspected children, we may see how teachers' rather nuanced roles with respect to ADHD play a significant part in medicalizing childhood deviance. Crucial here is the analysis of the familiarity teachers have with the diagnostic criteria for ADHD and how those are used as a framework in drawing up preliminary medical assessments of children suspected of having the disorder.

All but eight of the teachers I spoke with had no familiarity with *DSM IV*. The fact that so many of the teachers who so often suspect ADHD have no familiarity with *DSM IV* raises the question of what informs their diagnostic role in the classroom. The vast majority of respondents had no familiarity with the APA's official categorization for ADHD and yet were still integral agents in the process of suspecting and diagnosing the disorder. If the process of ADHD suspicion is alive and well within the classroom, yet is not informed by the nomenclature that has given ADHD its name, from where do these suspicions arise? An approach to this question might include addressing the different levels at which ADHD is suspected—and consequently invoked—within the school context. We may state that many teachers raise a flag of suspicion that promotes the more detailed labeling mechanisms within the school. Suspicion, therefore, need not begin with a particular nomenclature. Rather, suspicion begins in an unsophisticated way, in response to an unidentifiable trouble that may later become medically understood.

Testimony from teachers who understand and/or use *DSM IV* ADHD criteria reflect the influence psychiatric nomenclature has in defining childhood behavior in the classroom. One teacher, in a way minimizing her role as someone in the diagnostic process of ADHD, states: "Yeah, I'm aware of it, but that's more of a medical issue. I look for kids who are having problems, and even though I may suspect that a kid has ADHD, I'm not going to state it like I have made a diagnosis" (sixth and seventh grade teacher, age thirty-six). Suspecting ADHD is often influenced by the nomenclature of *DSM IV;* however, the use of the word *ADHD* is left up to others with the legitimate authority to make such medical declarations. ADHD as a medical category influences the process of how a child is being perceived in the classroom, but restraint is apparently exercised when presenting these suspicions in a definitive way. Refraining from stating *ADHD* delineates the nonmedical role teachers perceive themselves to occupy.

Other teachers express that having knowledge of *DSM IV* criteria is an important element in informing parents about their child's condition. As one respondent states: "Yeah, I have read those criteria. We had it handed out at a 'pro d' day two years ago. We refer to it once in a while especially when parents are in denial or are really defensive about their kids' problems" (seventh grade teacher, age forty-four). Illustrating the perceived necessity of developing a sound case for ADHD before informing parents of the team's conclusion, specific knowledge of *DSM IV* some teachers see as important in relieving parent defensiveness. Parental "denial," it is argued, can be alleviated when a child's behaviors are presented against the backdrop of *DSM IV* criteria. Teacher awareness of *DSM IV* is believed to be an important component of the efficacy of the school's recommendations. It is argued that in order for parents to be more accepting of a teacher or school recommendation, the invocation of some type of medical label for their child is crucial.

Respondents also state that knowledge of *DSM IV* criteria for ADHD can assist in the way schools deal with a suspected case of the disorder. As one teacher states: "Yes, I am (familiar with *DSM IV* criteria for ADHD). I don't give a diagnosis, but if I think a child may be wrongly diagnosed I will bring that up...Because I understand the *DSM* criteria OK, I can sometimes identify the problems" (special education teacher, age thirty-two). Such responses reveal the perception that teachers who are informed about *DSM IV* and utilize this diagnostic clarification effectively can influence the channels explored by the school as well as the recommendations that are made to parents. Here a reflexive relationship between teacher and the discipline structure of the school can be seen. In contrast to teachers who refrain from using the ADHD label, teachers can also play a role akin to a diagnostician. This appears paradoxical when teachers do not "give a diagnosis," yet use knowledge of *DSM IV* to influence the ways schools intervene with parents.

Making "the Case" for ADHD

The process of how school representatives suspect that a child may have ADHD manifests in many ways. Initially, teachers may simply make mental notes of a student they suspect as having a more significant struggle with assignments or behavioral control than other students. Teachers may see how a particular student stands out against his/her peers and relate what they see to previous knowledge about the ADHD condition. Depending upon the knowledge and experience of the teacher, the interpretation of a student's difficulties may vary widely. However, in dealing with excessively troublesome students, and an inevitable consultation with their parents, the process of suspicion becomes more formalized and may involve parties who meet in an effort to definitively label a given student's problems. These parties, who formulate what is known as a school-based team (SBT), may include the current and previous teacher of the student, a school psychologist, the principal (especially in disciplinary cases), and in instances when ADHD or other mental disorder is suspected, a medical professional, either a psychiatrist or perhaps a pediatrician. SBT meetings are typified by a discussion of a student's disciplinary and/or academic struggles, ultimately drawing inferences about the cause of these difficulties. In cases in which ADHD may be suspected, it is not uncommon for the SBT to refer directly to *DSM IV* criteria. The common results of such meetings include the development of what are called individualized education plans (IEPs) for troubled students and, in cases of suspected ADHD, a preliminary label of "probable ADHD." Both the development of education plans and the initial assessments that point to ADHD are later presented to parents. The initial meetings of the SBT and consequent conferences with parents are perhaps the most significant mechanism for suspecting ADHD children and ultimately moving them toward a formal, medical diagnosis.

Exemplified by the work of Georgia Burnley (1993), the approach to this method of identifying ADHD is based on a six-phase procedure: 1) preliminary assessment; 2) initial child-study team meeting; 3) formal assessment; 4) follow-up meeting of team; 5) collaborative meeting for strategy development; and 6) follow-up meetings and progress review (Burnley 1993, 228-30). Observations of the child presented at these meetings begin the larger machinery of the ADHD-assessment process. Therefore, it is believed that doctors or other mental health professionals should be privy to the information gathered by the school to make the

assessment process more effective. This sharing of information is corroborated by the clinician accounts we have examined previously.

Described by teachers as the standard method of intervention in cases
of ADHD, the SBT is a documentation of the phases of the transition
from informal to formal suspicion, culminating in pedagogical changes
designed to suit the needs of the ADHD student. The "preliminary assessment" denotes a team-building phase in which clinically unsubstantiated suspicions are discussed with other school personnel. Within these
discussions stories are shared and patterns are established. Formal assessment begins when team members' discussions specifically implicate
a learning disability or mental disorder label. At this phase, children may
be asked to complete one or many attention or behavior disorder tests,
the results of which may solidify a formal assessment and move the child
down the path to medical intervention.

In enhancing the team approach to observing ADHD, Carol Dowdy
(1998) argues that the teacher's role should be expanded in a clinical capacity. The author argues that teachers should not be mere automatons,
informing a team about the events of their classroom, the antics of certain children, etc. Teachers, Dowdy argues, must have a degree of
knowledge of ADHD: "Every teacher should have access to a copy of
the...(*DSM IV*) criteria and should be trained in identifying the characteristics that may be manifested in the classroom" (33). Knowledge of
ADHD symptoms should be accompanied by a procedure for documenting these behaviors:

> When teachers observe that several of the *DSM IV* behaviors
> are characteristic of one student...they should begin to keep a
> two week behavioral observation log. The log should docu-
> ment the child's attention-deficit-like behaviors and the times
> during which the behaviors appear to be more intense, occur
> more frequently, or are of longer duration. The specific class-
> room activities should also be noted, including the academic
> task and the type of activity (33).

Documentation bolsters the in-school ADHD assessment: "If the
teacher's observations continue to reflect significant attention-deficit-like
behaviors the school district's referral process should be initiated. The
observation log should be attached to the referral" (33).

A documentation of behavior is an important component, many teachers convey, in confirming a suspected case of ADHD. The preliminary
discussions at an SBT meeting, where parents are absent, serve as a

preparation for the more pivotal meeting to which parents are invited. Such preliminary meetings serve the purpose of compiling information and developing a case to present to parents. As one respondent states: "We present the findings of our meeting to the parents and explain our concerns, and we recommend that the parent pursue it through medical channels if it's severe enough" (special education teacher, age forty-five). Such meetings with parents, many teachers argue, have potential to be counterproductive if inadequate or unconvincing evidence is presented. Teachers state that parents are inclined to be very defensive about the mental states of their children and might quickly dismiss unwarranted opinions of the school. The SBT meetings, it is repeatedly argued, are places where a preliminary assessment of a child must be refined enough to prompt a convincing argument to the parents:

> I bring it (the possibility of a child having ADHD) up at an SBT meeting. From there we go in a lot of directions, but we usually bring the parents in to talk over some of the things we have been seeing and documenting. It's become really important that parents come in and know that we have been closely watching their child, otherwise they're likely to blow us off and not get any kind of medical intervention (fifth, sixth and seventh grade teacher, age forty).

As stated, the end goal with much of the SBT meetings surrounding ADHD is for parents to begin some process of medical intervention. Without a solid case, members of the SBT may be seen by parents as incompetent or unqualified to make medical recommendations. Therefore, the case for ADHD must be presented in as thorough and formal a manner as possible without giving the perception that the SBT is inappropriately practicing medicine.

As the SBT presents its case through psychiatric nomenclature, we see a median point within the informal/formal suspicion dichotomy established by Erving Goffman (1961) in his classic discussion of how mental patients become institutionalized. Because the SBT uses the language and diagnostic criteria of *DSM IV* and recommends assessments specifically for ADHD, we may be inclined to conclude that the SBT has many attributes characteristic of formal realms of mental health diagnoses. However, despite its continued use of clinical language and diagnostic tools, the school does not have the legitimate power to make formal declarations about the mental states of problem children. The school is an institution that acts as an intermediary between the lay world and the medical world. Because of this status, it might be more appropriate to examine the school, and more particularly the SBT, as a realm of "semi-formal," rather than formal, suspicion.

Though no uniform neurological perspective can be gleaned from the teachers I have interviewed, the strong influence of neurology can be seen in the ways in which teachers suspect ADHD children in their class-rooms, the types of ADHD intervention strategies they implement, and in the general way ADHD children are conceptualized.

The predominant characterization of ADHD children having "on-task" behavior problems shows a close fit between teachers' own classroom experiences and the neurologically oriented description of ADHD found in *DSM IV*. One teacher's description of ADHD children as suffering from "erratic impulses" exemplifies such a perspective. Despite a consis-tent invocation of clinical perspectives on ADHD, very few teachers had heard of or had any use for *DSM IV*. This reveals at least two coexisting possibilities about the ways clinical perspectives on ADHD influence the way people deal with and conceptualize the disorder. First, there is the possibility that teachers' perceptions of ADHD children match the *DSM IV* criteria because there is a strong fit between these diagnostic criteria and the way ADHD symptoms are manifested in the classroom. This says a considerable amount about the match between *DSM IV* criteria and the actual experience of teachers. It may be redundant for teachers to become familiar with *DSM IV* as their own experiences are the actual basis for *DSM IV* criteria. Second, there is also the possibility that teach-ers who deal with ADHD students (I would assume these to be most, if not all, teachers) spend enough time interacting with people (e.g., doctors and guidance counselors) who are influenced by clinical perspectives on the disorder that these perspectives shape teachers' experiences.

In being "semi-formal" in the way they suspect ADHD children, teachers operate in a hybridized lay and clinical role. Playing one part of this role, teachers witness rule breaking by certain students. It can be as-sumed that a good portion of such rule breaking is transitory and quickly normalized (Scheff 1999). In the instances in which this rule breaking is not remedied, teachers appeal to more informed parties, that is, those with expertise in diagnosing problems not remedied through normalizing measures. Enter the role of the SBT, a collection of people whose func-tion is to provide a crystallized definition of the child's problems, and in doing so, provide a path for the rectification of such problems. Often the SBT will solicit the opinions of medical experts, such as psychiatrists or pediatricians. At the point of implementing strategies advised by the

SBT, teachers become a part of the diagnostic and treatment process. Teachers are requested to begin a more rigorous documentation of the child, listing his/her infractions, having the child fill out questionnaires, and so on.

It is a matter of course that the more teachers witness disruptive behavior and the more they participate in SBT assessments of unruly children, the more they will become familiar with the signs attributed to ADHD. Hence, teachers with considerable experience in dealing with disruptive children may be able to inform parents about how a particular child fits a profile they have "seen before." This increasing familiarity is not necessitated by an expert understanding of *DSM IV* or any formal clinical experience. Teachers' increasing familiarity with ADHD results from knowledge being passed down from experts, primarily those who reside on the SBT. Such a transfer of knowledge perpetuates clinical perspectives on ADHD, greatly influencing the way teachers view these students and the way teachers raise suspicions of such students to parents.

In drawing parents' attention to problems with their children, teachers are in a precarious place. By presenting their case to parents too definitively ("I think your child has ADHD"), teachers risk appearing hasty in their generalizations. In addition, teachers also risk the appearance that they are overstepping their professional bounds. The "defensiveness" from parents many teacher respondents describe can be understood as a response to conclusions about their children that are seen as professionally inappropriate. Recalling previous testimony, some clinicians also feel that teachers need to focus on teaching instead of providing diagnoses. In order to express suspicion of ADHD, and not appear too convicting in the eyes of parents, or too encroaching upon clinicians' professional territory, teachers appeal to established ADHD knowledge, but not in an explicitly clinical manner.

This balancing act is partially achieved with the aid of the SBT and the case they build before presenting their suspicions of ADHD to parents. After the considerable documentation of infractions and after consultation with a mental health practitioner who can corroborate these suspicions, the SBT, the teacher, and the parents have a meeting in which these concerns are expressed. More often than not, these concerns are expressed through clinical language: parents are told that ADHD is an entrenched condition, that it is not their fault, and that it is treatable through medication.

Chapter Six

Responding to ADHD: School Curricula, Simplified Assignments, and Gender

Similar to the ways in which clinicians negotiate diagnostic and treatment protocols for ADHD, teachers negotiate between their professional concerns about the disorder and the bureaucratic structure of schools. Teachers unequivocally frame ADHD as an impediment to learning and therefore implicate ADHD in the frustration such students feel and the consequent disruptive behavior they demonstrate. Perhaps more so than anyone else, teachers witness the daily academic and social problems ADHD students encounter. As the interviews excerpted in this chapter illustrate, teachers own a high degree of agency in how they address ADHD children, particularly how they adapt school curricula to the perceived needs of such children. These curricular adaptations demonstrate the over-arching "master frame" teachers use to understand ADHD children, namely, that ADHD, whether neurological or environmental, induces behaviors that are outside of a child's control.

As will be shown, teachers contend that the single most important professional response to ADHD children in their classrooms is to take whatever steps are necessary to make them feel a sense of connection to their academic pursuits, consequently making the classroom a less threatening environment. This includes the simplification of assignments, making allowances for certain types of behavior, allowing assignments to be completed in smaller bits, and so on. Interestingly, none of the teachers I interviewed contend, that their school or school district had specific pedagogical protocols that were to be followed for children with ADHD. Hence, when it comes to addressing ADHD, teachers exercise a considerable amount of freedom in the measures they employ. Aside from the modification of assignments, teachers conveyed varied opinions of the effectiveness of labeling a child as having ADHD and also offered considerable discussion about how the disciplinary standards of school curricula contribute to the "gendering" of the disorder.

Classroom Connectedness and the Prevention of Deviance

As ADHD children are perceived to be mentally different, it follows that the majority of teachers adopt certain strategies to accommodate such children in the learning environment. The nature of different teaching strategies provides insight into how teachers see the inner nature of ADHD children. When addressing what teaching techniques they employ to educate children with ADHD, teachers revealed more about how they frame ADHD children, more specifically, how they perceive their learning capabilities, their fit with school curricula, and their long-term prognosis for learning. The most common accommodation concerns the modification of assignments. As ADHD children are framed as oppositional toward and easily ignored by school curricula, teachers argue that such modification is important for cultivating a sense of connectedness, in which the small successes of easier assignments create confidence in learning. Teachers also point out that the employment of such methods for teaching ADHD children should not overshadow the use of generally effective teaching methods. Though assignments could be, and in many cases *must* be modified in the case of ADHD, many teachers feel that being an overall solid facilitator of learning is equally important.

ADHD and the Urgency of Intervention

Intervention strategies, it is repeatedly argued, need to be done early in a child's school career to adequately deal with the ADHD condition. According to many teachers, the negative symptoms of untreated ADHD become more ingrained as children grow older. Teachers argue that a student first diagnosed with ADHD in high school, for example, has a lessened chance of living a normal life than, say, a child diagnosed in second grade. The undiscovered or forgotten student with ADHD is perceived as highly vulnerable, what many teachers call "at-risk." A failure to treat ADHD would lead to shortcomings in an ADHD child's base of knowledge and ability to reason. Often referred to as "holes" or "gaps," these shortcomings are argued to compound, eventually compromising an ADHD student's future. One teacher describes this:

> They're sharp, but they may have some holes in their learning. They are getting a fragmented education, missing certain skills. ...They may drop out of school and not continue any

kind of education. Then there's all kinds of stuff waiting for them. One boy I had and his parents were really afraid of medication, that it would be addictive and get him into other drugs. I told him, 'This will not get you into drugs. This will keep you away from drugs' (fourth, fifth and sixth grade teacher, age forty-two).

Shortcomings in academic skills, it is argued, eventually impede the comprehension of increasingly complicated school lessons. While normal children, according to some respondents, are "learning how to learn," ADHD children paint themselves into an intellectual corner. "Holes" in an ADHD child's learning will persist and multiply until they make continuation in school impossible. By expressing to parents that the use of medication prevents children from taking illicit drugs, this teacher implies that such measures are integral to academic success and avoidance of self-destructive behaviors that arise when educational opportunities are squandered. Failing such a connection to school, it is argued, ADHD children who do not achieve some degree of academic success become susceptible to engaging in deviant lifestyles. As one teacher states:

> Without treatment I think a case of ADHD can be really tragic. The last thing someone with untreated ADHD wants to do is go to school. Without school you just don't have a lot of options like you used to have. You can't even learn a trade without a high school diploma. It can really be tragic...taking drugs. Without school there isn't a lot else to put your energy into (special education teacher, age fifty-five).

And another teacher:

> If that kid's need goes unmet in school then you can have all sorts of problems later in life. Where else are they going to go? Where are they going to get job skills? If we lose them here, its going to be a long hard road. Once they get isolated from other kids who are going somewhere, they become susceptible to all sorts of things, like gangs, drugs, all of it (fourth grade teacher, age fifty-one).

Other teachers mentioned that success in school is a way to protect would-be vulnerable children from predatory types of people. One teacher referred to these persons as "recruiters":

I'm afraid they can become very antisocial and drop out of school. This really puts them at risk for the social ills that are out there. These kids will rely on being cool, rather than fitting into the system and having success in it. ...Recruiters prey upon that, take advantage of these kids who have given up on themselves (special education teacher, age fifty-two).

ADHD children, it is argued, may give up on the academic components of school and instead focus on the informal aspects of that environment: being cool, acting tough, and so on. Teachers contend that ADHD children who lose their academic footing are more easily influenced by representatives of deviant lifestyles. The teacher from whom this passage comes also tells the story of a sixth grade girl who was diagnosed with ADHD and never treated. At fifteen or sixteen years of age she dabbled in drugs and eventually dropped out of high school. On his way home from work, this teacher saw her in a "skid row" area engaging in what appeared to be prostitution. He has not seen her since and has no idea of what ultimately became of her.

Modifying Assignments

The majority of teachers state that they alter their approaches to ADHD children by shortening the length of assignments so that such children could complete at least some of the tasks at hand. As one teacher states: "I guess I try to make sure the activities are a little bit shorter than normal. If I notice a child beginning to get restless, I try and break things up a little bit, if I can. In smaller chunks these children can do pretty good" (fifth and sixth grade teacher, age forty-six). Such augmentation of assignments is said to cultivate a sense of accomplishment for ADHD children and make them feel more a part of the classroom: "I use shortened assignments to enable them to get a sense of success. I also like to give choices in what the kids are able to do. They don't have to do the things in order if they don't want to" (second and third grade teacher, age forty-seven).

From a psychodynamic perspective, ADHD symptoms are often perceived to be a reaction to a world that seems to misunderstand or is unsympathetic to the special condition of ADHD children. What appears to be impulse-driven behavior, from this perspective, is really an expression of frustration children have in dealing with the conventions of everyday life. The modification of assignments on behalf of teachers is meant to relieve the frustration believed to cripple children with ADHD. By modifying assignments and breaking them into smaller, more digestible pieces, teachers try to relieve the negative associations ADHD children may make with the classroom.

In accommodating ADHD children and removing negativity from the classroom, teachers also state that it is important to acknowledge that ADHD children have an inclination for unconventional classroom behavior and that this is not to be entirely discouraged. As one teacher states: "It's also really important to let these kids work with other kids, you know, work a little, talk a little. I try not to be draconian when it comes to the kids because I think they really need to talk sometimes. Giving them motion and movement is also really important" (second and third grade teacher, age forty-two). Another respondent allows the use of CD players as they are perceived to help ADHD children focus: "I'm also not opposed to allowing the kids to wear headphones (CD players) while they're working. The ADHD kids just settle right down once they get the headphones on" (special education teacher, age forty-three). Such responses demonstrate that teachers are flexible in dealing with such children. Instead of the schools being perceived as an unyielding, rigid institution, responses that describe alterations in the curriculum or allowances in behavior demonstrate that the school attempts to address ADHD through its own internal adjustments. However, in response to these adjustments it may be pertinent to ask whether or not the creation of a sense of success is done at the expense of curriculum quality. Does the reduction in expected workload of ADHD children keep them involved with the pedagogical process, or does it further separate these children from others? By lowering academic expectations, teachers contend that making schoolwork more inviting to ADHD children is an acceptable trade-off if it cultivates greater cohesion between such students and the classroom.

The Special Geography of ADHD Learners

A considerable number of respondents state that teaching techniques for ADHD are best implemented in more learning-intensive environments in which children with distractibility problems and extreme learning difficulties can receive more one-on-one attention. Special Education or Learning Assistance Center (LAC) classrooms[1] are places where the special needs of ADHD children and others with learning problems could be accommodated. Invariably, the design of the centers I visited was similar in two significant ways.

First, all of the LACs I examined were considerably small compared to a conventional classroom. It would be difficult to accommodate more than a dozen students in one LAC at one time. Because of this reduced size there is potential for a tremendous amount of direct teacher-to-student interaction—something believed to specifically address the needs of ADHD children. One LAC reveals a semicircle of tiny chairs that are oriented toward the chalkboard; the chair closest to the board facing outward is for the teacher. The teacher I was interviewing sat in the tiny chair and demonstrated to me how he does a lesson. Remarkable about the orientation of the chairs and the design of the room was the degree of intimacy such conditions cultivated. In accordance with some of the neurological postulates about ADHD children, the LAC fosters a pervasive reinforcement of school lessons. Such reinforcement comes not through an occasional reminder to get "back on task" but occurs through a constant teacher presence.

Second, the LACs had a "no frills" decor that appeared very controlled and, frankly, rather drab. One could not help but feel a lack of conventional classroom items. Mobiles hanging from the ceiling, colorful paintings on the walls, cartoons that advocate learning, all of these were omitted from the design of the room. Lessons were neatly stacked along some bookcases on either side of the room, perfectly organized and accessible. The absence of superfluous items was justified as part of a teaching technique that sought a minimum of outside distractions and also as a way of avoiding the display of children's completed projects that would cultivate a sense of competition and bitterness among them. With the absence of such items, the decor of the LAC combines psychodynamic and neurological perspectives on ADHD. From the neurological stance, minimizing distractions is an obvious way to control the stimuli that ADHD children receive in the learning environment, therefore aiding them in focusing on their work. In accommodating psychodynamic mandates about ADHD, the reduction in competitiveness that stems from not displaying children's work makes the environment less belittling for kids who strongly associate school with failure.

The Lack of School Consensus Regarding ADHD

In addressing the pedagogical needs attributed to difficult and "potentially ADHD" children, many teachers claim that their primary purpose is to rigorously meet the expectations that define their profession. As many teachers discuss, the lack of specified school protocols for ADHD students leaves teachers the option of "doing what they do best." As one respondent states: "For me, it's really about being an effective teacher. I haven't seen any kind of protocol for ADHD kids in our school or from the district" (seventh grade teacher, age forty). As it is presented at professional development workshops on ADHD the model of the ideal "ADHD teacher" does not really address the specifics of ADHD, but instead describes an overall pedagogical competence. During the workshops I attended, the "techniques" for teaching ADHD children included: (1) Being specific in the directions you give; (2) Giving notification well in advance of any upcoming work that may require extended effort; and (3) Spending more one-on-one time with ADHD students, if possible. In talking with teachers, it appears that many feel these kinds of recommendations are strategies applicable to *all* students, not just those with ADHD. These informal comments imply that "ADHD protocols" are not developed because the methods prescribed to teach ADHD children are already used by any competent teacher.

In being asked to specifically accommodate ADHD children, many teachers state that they are essentially being asked to become even *more* effective—a task considered by one teacher to be daunting:

> I think just solid teaching is what needs to be done for these kids, but that's tougher these days with the increase in class sizes that have been occurring. I don't really know of any techniques that we use to just teach ADHD kids, other than being present and taking part in giving them attention and care (sixth and seventh grade teacher, age fifty).

Addressed in this excerpt is the issue of structural constraints encroaching upon the profession of teaching. Teachers also argue that solid teaching for ADHD and non-ADHD children is more difficult given the increasing demands placed upon teachers. Interestingly, even though a few respondents mention class size as an impediment to providing effective teaching strategies, no respondents allude to the idea that increases in class size affect the extent to which children in the classroom may act out and hence become suspected of having ADHD. In short, no teachers I interviewed drew a linkage between increased class size and increases in ADHD diagnoses.

The fact that there are few ADHD teaching protocols speaks again to the perceptions of what constitutes ADHD and whether or not ADHD is a valid diagnostic category. Unlike learning impediments, such as dyslexia, dysgraphia, or other problems in which there are specific teaching protocols, ADHD, according to teachers, remains largely unrecognized. This lack of recognition stems from at least two factors. First, ADHD symptomatology represents such a plethora of behaviors that the establishment of one teaching protocol is highly problematic. Accommodations for students with problems focusing and completing their work are perceived by many teachers to be "part of the job." Second, ADHD symptoms, such as impulsivity and lack of focus, are behaviors expected of children. Most children surely experience restlessness or academic struggle from time to time, but determining when these instances represent ADHD or not remains highly subjective. Therefore, the distinction between the times when a teacher adopts an aggressive yet conventional approach to a troubled student and when a teacher employs teaching strategies for a "disordered" student is difficult to make.

For many respondents the lack of consensus within the school is equated to a kind of child neglect. The school, it is argued, fails to accommodate children with ADHD through its curriculum design. As one respondent states: "It's a question of do you force the student or do you adapt the curriculum, and I don't think we have sorted that out yet" (seventh grade teacher, age thirty-two). The failure to provide the needed structure for ADHD children puts such children at an increased risk for academic hardship, many teachers argue. For example, when asked whether or not he feels his school had a consensus on how to deal with ADHD children, one teacher states: "No, not at all, and it's a big problem. You get a kid who might have a bad mental problem, and no one knows what to do when he gets into a later grade and starts having problems" (special education teacher, age forty-four). This excerpt demonstrates a previous theme that schools must begin the process of identification and accommodation earlier when it comes to ADHD children and certainly speaks to the argument that teachers need to have a greater awareness of what constitutes ADHD. Also implied here is that when older students begin to demonstrate severe learning problems, there is no comprehensive intervention program within the curriculum. Hence, the lack of consensus that impedes early intervention becomes increasingly problematic as the child gets older and encounters a more challenging workload. Because there is no protocol for dealing with all of the manifestations of ADHD (i.e., social, academic, disciplinary, and so on), it is argued that students will fall through the cracks.

The lack of consensus is also attributed to a void in teacher understandings of ADHD symptoms. As one teacher remarks, the difference between times when a child is making normal adjustments versus the times when he/she is demonstrating ADHD symptoms remains unclear: "What if a kid is just having a bad day or a bad month? Do we just put him in remedial classes and recommend that he be medicated?" (special education teacher, age forty-four). The issue here concerns the interpretation of childhood misbehavior. At what point, this teacher's questions imply, do schools determine that a child's misbehavior is in fact pathological? Further, when the determination is made that the behavior might be ADHD and warrants medical treatment, what is the basis of such a determination?

Teachers also contend that some of their colleagues spend too much time focusing on issues of hyperactivity rather than the cognitive manifestations of ADHD. As one teacher states: "We focus way too much on the hyperactivity criteria rather than the ADD criteria. With those kids the mind is all over the place, rather than the body. Teachers tend to focus on the physically active kids, and that's a mistake" (special education teacher, age forty-two). The mind of the inattentive case of ADHD is ignored because of the very visible and disturbing behaviors exhibited by students who are more easily labeled "hyperactive." This emphasis on behavior rather than academic failure as a sign of possible ADHD is no doubt a factor in teacher support of medical intervention through the administration of stimulant medications. Hyperactivity, it is argued, can be greatly reduced once a trial of Ritalin begins, and this verifies that the teacher's suspicion was correct in the first instance.

Teachers' perceived causes of disruptive classroom behavior are also placed into question. For many teachers who believe that misbehavior is symptomatic of ADHD, their schools are a place laden with those who refuse to see such behavior in the same way. As one teacher says: "Today we still have a lot of disbelievers, you know, 'spare the rod' kind of thinking" (sixth and seventh grade teacher, age fifty). Such "disbelievers" are argued to be an impediment to constructing a schoolwide consensus toward ADHD. Their colleagues contend that these teachers view behavioral problems in a manner that defies a lot of the neurological positions about misbehavior and ADHD. Instead of interpreting overt hyperactive behavior as originating from a neurological dysfunction, respondents argue that some of their colleagues anachronistically view these problems as character defects, rectified through traditional disciplinary avenues.

The lack of school consensus in dealing with ADHD also reflects the nature of past and current ADHD discussions. Aside from the criteria provided by *DSM IV*—criteria that remain shrouded in skepticism—there is no unifying mode for a diagnosis of ADHD. The attitudes of teachers towards ADHD are indeed a reflection of this state of ADHD discourse. For some teachers, the "class clown" has not changed and requires no deeper examination: certain kids act up; and these kids need to be held accountable for their behavior. For others, the discourse of ADHD has shed new light on what prompts some children to misbehave.

The issue of school consensus is further complicated by the wide range of behaviors that comprise ADHD. In interpreting kids' severe academic problems, teachers are more inclined to link these problems to learning disabilities or dyslexia than to ADHD. As the description of the difference between ADHD and non-ADHD students demonstrates, the ADHD label is almost exclusively pinned on the kids who misbehave, as opposed to those who have academic problems. In this sense, the diagnosis of ADHD—one that most often pathologizes disciplinary and academic problems—is a poison pill for some teachers to swallow. Subscribing to the ADHD diagnosis partially justifies weakness in the curriculum and impedes the maintenance of disciplinary and academic standards.

The bureaucratic reception of ADHD that de facto dismisses the existence of the disorder is, according to some teachers, part of a larger issue of rigidity in the public education system. For many teachers the simple matter is that different learning styles are not recognized, and if protocols for different styles of learning did exist, they would be impossible to implement because of increasing class size. As one respondent states: "It's really hard to try to implement anything that's just for one type of learner. And if we were asked to do that, we would probably have to double our staff." (sixth and seventh grade teacher, age thirty-six). Hence, not accommodating ADHD students is connected to the recurring problem of the perceived invalidity of the ADHD diagnosis and the fact that there are not the staff resources available to employ effective techniques even if a diagnosis of ADHD is given more institutional legitimacy.

As demonstrated, ADHD has never had a history of being an elegant category of illness. Because of the gelatinous nature of ADHD's symptoms, the cause of the disorder has had various interpreters, many of whom vehemently dispute the adequacy of other perspectives. Despite the prevailing dominance of neurology in framing ADHD, the disorder remains shrouded in popular and academic debate. The diagnosis, many critics contend, remains highly subjective, its ultimate impact on our culture ambiguous. At the level of education policy, where the most cutting-edge research remains largely unintelligible and irrelevant, the ambiguity of ADHD is strongly preserved. Until ADHD becomes categorically recognized as a bona fide learning impediment in public schools—a time, many may argue, that will never arrive until the disorder's legitimacy can be firmly established—it seems unlikely that teachers will implement significant and consistent changes in school curricula.

Negotiating the Impact of the ADHD Label

As with other medical conditions, especially those associated with mental health, ADHD, despite the wide variety in its symptomatology, is a diagnosis with social consequences. One such consequence stems from the fact that ADHD has a meaning in social life that affects and constructs personal identity of the labeled person and influences his/her social interaction. Due to teachers' significance in suspecting ADHD, and hence applying the ADHD label to children, it was important to solicit responses from teachers regarding their opinions on the ADHD label and its impact on children. In discussing the social circumstances that may result from a child's being labeled as having ADHD, teachers offer a range of opinions, though most subscribe to the idea that the ADHD label, once given, remains a relatively permanent fixture throughout a child's life. A significant theme in the interviews with teachers concerns the dangerousness of the ADHD label's social-psychological permanency. For others, the ADHD label, if given correctly and mediated responsibly, is argued to be beneficial in that it serves as a reminder that ADHD will always be present in the diagnosed person's life.

Teachers who express concern over the process of labeling a child ADHD commonly give opinions that resonate with many of the positions established in sociological studies of deviance. Within these responses are concerns over the fact that labels, especially those that concern a mental health diagnosis, have a permanent quality:

> Once labeled it travels with them everywhere. That's a big
> concern that I have. Once they get a [diagnosis] as LD [learn-
> ing disability]—which is really ADHD for a lot of these
> kids—they will always see themselves that way. Maybe in the
> short run it's OK, but down the road that has got to affect self-
> esteem (sixth grade teacher, age fifty-five).

In stating that the ADHD label "travels with them everywhere," this
teacher is highlighting significant contributions from labeling theory in
sociology (Rosenhan 1973). Within this facet of sociology, the social
manifestations of a label are not restricted to institutional contexts. The
diagnosis of ADHD, for example, affects not only the way a child is
taught, but also the way in which he/she is perceived in everyday life.
There is, in effect, a significant social-psychological relationship between the labeled individual and his/her surroundings in which the contents of the label become more widely known to larger social networks
and prompt interactions that are filtered through the label's meaning.
This culminates in changes in the identity of the child—changes that
many sociologists and psychologists argue are difficult to reverse.

Strongly implied by these types of concerns over the ADHD label are
the way shifts in personal identity foster a process of social ostracism.
These issues were highlighted in Edwin Lemert's (1962) famous essay,
"Paranoia and the Dynamics of Exclusion." Within the process Lemert
characterized as "the generic process of exclusion," persons who had
acquired some type of deviant identity were slowly pushed away from
mainstream life. Two crucial elements of this process include: 1) an increasing tendency for the interactions between the labeled individual and
the social group to become more shallow in nature; and 2) a lack of fit
between the affect of the "exclusionary group" and the attitudes this
group carries about the labeled person.

Interactions between the labeled person and the exclusionary group
become more spurious as the status of the deviant individual is perceived
to be a dominant part of his/her character. In the case of mental disorder
labels, interactions become superficial because the larger social group
collectively feels that the deviant person is socially incompetent. Justified by the notion that the deviant label must have originated from
somewhere and therefore is valid, this assumption of incompetence ultimately affects the way in which the labeled person imagines how he is
being perceived.

According to Lemert, the labeled individual rightfully assumes that
there is a different perception of him/herself than the image conveyed

through symbolic exchanges between him/herself and the larger social group. The group's affect has become more "small talk" and patronizing, and this prompts the labeled person to attempt to rectify the discrepancy. He/she becomes confrontational, demanding that the group give up the information and reveal what they are really thinking and why. Unaware that their own attitude shifts have caused this confrontational behavior, the group interprets such confrontations as further signs of mental disorder. Thus, a vicious cycle of interaction ensues in which the deviant individual becomes increasingly paranoid and further detached from those who used to provide a stable component to the social-psychological process of "normal" identity.

Lemert's discussion of the dynamics between excluded individual and exclusionary group are rooted in his theoretical positions about the progressive stages of deviance, especially his notion of "secondary deviation." At this phase of social deviance, the individual, having been rejected by mainstream society, fully adopts a deviant identity and seeks others with similar social status. Persons with a mainstream identity become foreign to the deviant, and reintegration into normal society a shrinking possibility. This move into a solidified deviant identity is attributed to social dynamics rather than to individual behavior. The deviant is effectively forced into a deviant lifestyle because the greater community refuses to allow that person to reintegrate.

Teacher concerns over the ADHD label demonstrate a social sensitivity to the effects of labels and prompt an inquiry into the extent to which the ADHD label may create circumstances similar to those Lemert describes. Within the confines of school there are myriad social situations, the dynamics of which certainly will be influenced by the meaning of the ADHD label. Situations such as a child's being absent from regular class to attend a session at an LAC is one of many examples. It is logical that other kids will wonder why one student is being treated differently, why assignments seem to be modified for particular students, and so on. The children asking about the ones who are being specially treated may formulate a type of exclusionary group that develops judgments about that child's character. Such judgments could drastically alter the course of the ADHD child's social life.

The child's "ADHD social identity" could also be inaccurate, according to many teachers. Familiar with the recurring issue of ADHD diagnostic validity and reliability, many teachers argue that the ADHD label, if given incorrectly, obscures attention to some of the child's more significant circumstances. As one teacher states:

> Three years ago we had one kid who was severely LD, and he
> also was taking meds for his hyperactivity. We met with his
> mom and found out that his stepfather was supposedly beating
> him. So they're medicating this kid, and there is this major
> problem at home with probable child abuse. They're totally
> ignoring this kid, and they could have given him a label that
> would have helped his situation rather than avoiding it (sev-
> enth grade teacher, age thirty-two).

Pertinent here are issues of accuracy in the identification of childhood
trauma. In the instance of a child who was likely being abused at home
and acting out his home-life frustrations at school, medication is argued
to be an incorrect, if not inhumane, choice. By quashing behavioral problems more attributable to external family dynamics than to internal neurological or psychological problems, medication only places a veneer on
the child's actual troubles. Another teacher expresses a similar concern
about the application of the ADHD label in lieu of an examination of
family struggles:

> If the label is incorrect—and I think it can be—there could be
> some real problems. I would hate to think about a kid taking
> medication when there was really nothing wrong with him but
> that there was a problem with the family we all overlooked.
> You just have to be very thorough in dealing with trying to
> categorize the kid's behavior (fifth, sixth and seventh grade
> teacher, age forty).

The thoroughness recommended by this teacher seems problematic in
addressing some of the immediate behavioral problems perceived to represent ADHD. Because the child who acts up is believed to be sur-
rounded by crisis, action to alleviate the behavior is often taken immediately. In advocating a more exhaustive approach to exploring why a child
may act out or suffer academically, such teachers present the case for an
examination of the greater social world of the child before entertaining
the idea that the child's problems are medical in nature.

For other teachers, labeling a child as having ADHD is a concern because of the label's own volatility. Such teachers argue that care must be
taken in order to mediate the amount of knowledge people have about a
child's condition: "It (the label) should be kind of kept quiet. Other kids
can be pretty harsh when they know some other kid has a problem or has
to take meds or something like that. I think teachers need to try and con-

trol that a little bit" (special education teacher, age forty-three). Within the hands of other children, for example, the knowledge about one of their peers, having ADHD is perceived to be potentially damaging to the self-image of the labeled child. As stated, the responsibility for regulating this information rests upon the shoulders of adults, most especially teachers. It is also argued that knowledge about the ADHD label needs to be kept not only from the cruel grasp of other children but also from ADHD children themselves:

> With labeling you don't want the kid to know what label has been applied. You definitely want the parents and teachers to know so that they can be aware of what to do for the child, but the kid should be told that he is normal and OK (special education teacher, age fifty-two).

As a mental disorder label may damage self-image and foster a separation from mainstream life, the maintenance of a normal identity even throughout the suspicion and diagnosis process is argued to be integral to the psychological health of ADHD children. This implies a great deal of adult responsibility in mediating between the label of ADHD and those social forces that may respond harshly toward it. The adults who surround an ADHD child must be privy to the knowledge that the child has ADHD so that appropriate remedial measures can be taken, but it must be noted that additional measures include preventing ADHD children from feeling the judgments of the greater social world.

"If the Label Fits..."

As mediators of how the ADHD label is applied, teachers clearly express concern over the social ramifications of labeling and see themselves as integral social actors in softening the stigma for ADHD children. Contrary to such perspectives, other teachers in the respondent group said they did not have any major concerns about the process of labeling children ADHD. Such teachers contend that ADHD, if applied correctly, can be the beginnings of effective school-based treatment for the disorder. As one teacher states: "The label can be beneficial if it's the right one. We can get those kids the help they really need" (sixth and seventh grade teacher, age thirty-four). In the event of a correct diagnosis of ADHD it is argued that such children become more understood and better accommodated by pedagogical restructuring. Teachers also express the connection between the ADHD label and the necessity of medication: "It can be really helpful if you have the correct label and get the kid on the right kind of medication. The label helps us develop strategies to aid the kid in his learning" (fifth and sixth grade teacher, age forty-four). Such statements reveal a subscription to a combination of both medication use and teaching techniques to deal with ADHD. The label of ADHD, if made correctly, can prompt pharmacological attention and an alteration in classroom teaching strategies.

In specific contrast to teachers who argue that knowledge of the label of ADHD must be kept from the child, some teachers express that the ADHD label is necessary for adults to correctly understand ADHD children, and also for ADHD children to have greater self-understanding. As one teacher states:

> The label can also promote self-awareness. If people see the kid and know what he has, then they can treat him accordingly. The media discussion of medication I think has a lot to do with the fear of labels, but this kind of judgment can be detrimental (fourth, fifth and sixth grade teacher, age forty-two).

Chapters 3 and 4 illustrated the perception that ADHD children do not have a strong ability to reflect upon themselves and the ramifications of their behavior. They are, by this definition, impulsive. The ADHD label, it is argued, can be integral to the child's development of self-awareness and resistance to impulse. From the perspective of ADHD children and the adults who treat them, the ADHD label need not be a source of stigma. The diagnosis of ADHD is seen as correcting the relationship between ADHD children and the adult world that adopts responsibility for their treatment. In addition, this response also offers a commentary on the public perception of ADHD and medication. The public, it is implied, has fears about medication and ADHD, fears that can impede the process of identifying children with the disorder. The "detrimental" condition expressed by this passage denotes that impediments to identifying children with ADHD will disrupt intervention into the child's life until it may be too late for such strategies to be effective.

The ADHD Label and Gender

Mirroring academic discourse about the sex-based epidemiology of ADHD, numerous teachers' discussions reveal that labeling children ADHD is a gendered phenomenon. Given the fact that roughly one in ten ADHD children is female, it is not surprising that teachers unanimously claim that boys comprise most of the cases of ADHD in their classrooms. Perhaps more interesting is not the fact that teacher responses reflect the known gender breakdown of ADHD children but rather how the interpretations teachers offer explain why there would be a discrepancy between genders in the prevalence of ADHD. In offering these interpretations, teachers express a considerable sociological sensitivity, discussing how the gender socialization process relates to the visibility of the disorder, and also, how it is more difficult for boys to follow a school's disciplinary standards than it is for girls.

In offering a sociological commentary on ADHD and gender, teachers describe how goys and girls have different emotional and expressive needs and that these are the product of social forces. For example, when asked about the gender of her ADHD students, one teacher states :

> Definitely more males. Probably double the amount of girls, but I think we miss a lot of the girls. They are more emotionally needy, trained different. With boys its very visible, they act out externally. But the inattention with both is the same kind (special education teacher, age thirty-nine).

This passage epitomizes many of the responses that offer reasons for the gender discrepancy in cases of ADHD. There are two intertwined positions implicit here. First, girls have a different set of interactive needs from boys. They are framed as being more inclined to seek out emotional support, and therefore have a smaller propensity to engage in overtly antisocial behavior. Second, girls are not framed as being entirely exempt from the disorder; however, if they have ADHD, they are far less visible. Girls may in fact have the symptoms of ADHD (academic failure, socially inappropriate behavior, restlessness, and so on) but because their behaviors are less overt than the types of behavior exhibited by boys, they are not detected as readily.

The issue at the core of why there is such a huge gender discrepancy in instances of ADHD has more to do with behavioral visibility than with the actual existence of the condition. Much like the case of compulsion neuroses documented by Anna Freud, teachers contend that girls are said to manifest the disorder in an introverted fashion, acting spacey and dreamy: "With the girls they may just space out when it comes to getting their work done, but we don't usually say that that's a case of ADD or ADHD. Maybe people just expect that more of girls" (fifth and sixth grade teacher, age forty-four). From a psychoanalytic perspective, girls are disinclined to lash out at the outside world in moments of rapid cathexis. Teachers often attribute this difference to the process of socialization:

> I think it's a socialization thing. Girls are taught at a young age to not act out, to internalize their feelings. Boys are always taught to act out. I think that's why girls tend to have self-destructive problems when they get frustrated or upset. They haven't been taught to express themselves and get those feelings out. Boys tend to destroy the things that are outside of themselves, you know, externally (seventh grade teacher, age thirty-four).

The above excerpt suggests that the identification of ADHD may be a moment in which we see gender socialization. We may ask whether or not the suspicion of ADHD is linked to behaviors that are culturally expected from boys. Because they are socialized to externalize their emotions, boys may find themselves in more conflict with the external world. Rather than turn their frustrations inward, boys are perceived to alter the external world to their own specifications. That is, boys are socialized to avoid internal adjustments to difficulties with the world and are taught that the source of relief lies within making external changes.

Teachers also comment that the higher visibility of male ADHD cases may also be due to the restrictive behavioral expectations schools place upon their students. The institution of education, it is argued, remains intolerant of behaviors that we commonly associate with boyhood. As one teacher states:

> Public schools are not geared towards adolescent boys. We do not tolerate the things we most associate with them, like roughhousing, doing pranks, picking fights and all of that. Some of these things are clearly destructive, but some other things may not be so clear cut, like why is it always discouraged to talk out of turn? Maybe that's necessary for some boys' mental health (seventh grade teacher, age forty).

In *The War against Boys* (2000), a critique of how boyhood has become stigmatized and the subject of reform in public schools, Christina Hoff Sommers argues that behaviors we have traditionally labeled as "typically male" (*boys will be boys!*) are increasingly targeted as antisocial and unhealthy. In focusing a good part of her argument upon how public schools have become a proving ground for programs designed to resocialize boys into more passive, and hence more feminine, social roles, Hoff Sommers offers illuminating commentary on changes in the tolerance threshold of schools. Behavior that used to be met with strict disciplinary measures is now being understood as indicative of a systemic problem with the male gender; medicalization, therefore, is an increasingly gendered phenomenon.

In light of Hoff Sommers's work, we may ask about the extent to which antimale ideology fosters a greater intolerance toward young males. As a colleague of mine asked: "Isn't giving Ritalin the same as chemical castration?" In answering this, we may acknowledge that Hoff Sommers offers some compelling positions. In their disciplinary practices, schools encourage behaviors associated with female socialization: passiveness, quietness, obedience, and so on. Because of these behavioral expectations, the larger spectrum of adolescent behavior is not tolerated, and some parts of it highly discouraged. This also alludes to the possibility that the restrictive quality of the school might not adequately address the mental health needs of boys. As some teachers contend, perhaps talking out of turn is not a sign of mental disorder but is instead a mechanism for boys to ensure their own mental health.

Notes

1. For the sake of simplicity, I use the term *learning assistance center* generically. The numerous schools I visited had various titles for centers that were designed for children with learning and/or social difficulties.

Chapter Seven

Parents' Accounts: How Trouble Becomes ADHD

Our first examination of interviews with parents of ADHD children[1] analyzes how their children's intellectual and interpersonal problems precipitated suspicions of ADHD. Through examining accounts of these problems, this chapter employs the "Micro-Politics of Trouble" framework posited by Robert M. Emerson and Sheldon L. Messinger (1977) and substantiates how childhood troubles become "cooperatively" framed (Miller and Silverman 1995, 725) as signs of mental disorder. Demonstrated through parents' accounts, and corroborating the interview data examined in chapter 4, schools are the most common institutional context for the discovery of children's troubles that are believed to be indicative of ADHD, and schools are the most involved institutions in moving a case of suspected ADHD toward a formal medical diagnosis. By highlighting the connection between a child's troubles and the school, this chapter shows how the institutions of the family and the school are interconnected in the interpretation of childhood troubles and the transformation of such troubles into a discernible form of deviance.

As Emerson and Messinger (1977) describe, the process by which a trouble becomes normalized and forgotten or progressively interpreted as a specific form of deviance is directly related to the social organization of persons associated with the trouble. Summarizing this framework, the authors state that "the natural history of a trouble is intimately tied to—and produces—the effort to do something about it" (Emerson and Messinger 1977, 123). This perspective resonates with two mainstay sociology-of-deviance assertions: first, that we do not recognize deviance through the intrinsic nature of the deviant act but through the way people organize themselves and form a response to that act (Becker 1963), and second, that the communicative dynamics among parties constitutes the "interaction order" (Maynard 1988, 312) in relation to a developing notion of deviance.

As a more developed conceptual scheme of Erving Goffman's (1961) discussion of the differences between "informal" and "formal" suspicion in the diagnosis of the mentally ill, Emerson and Messinger (1977, 121) contend that the transformation of a trouble into a designated form of deviance can be seen through the trouble's discussion in "informal" and then "official" realms. In short, the authors argue that the failure of informal methods to correct troubles will prompt a mobilization of parties who implement remedial measures in an increasingly sophisticated manner. Official remediation marks the point at which troubles may become public knowledge and are formally labeled (Emerson and Messinger 1977, 128). Such labeling is, of course, very relevant in analyses of the medicalization of deviant behavior and, as the present chapter reveals, is particularly appropriate for the study of how adults frame children's troubles as medical phenomena.

The micropolitics-of-trouble framework has had significant empirical application in accounts of the social construction of social problems. Such studies include the analyses of work incentive programs (Miller 1983), self-help groups for persons with affective disorders (Karp 1992), and the identification of family abuse (Webster and O'Toole 1989). Aspects of the framework have also been applied to the analysis of social control with a specific application to the social control of children (Kivett and Warren 2002; McKeganey 1984). As this chapter will demonstrate, the micropolitics framework is also an excellent way to contextualize parents' and children's initial experiences with the problems that become framed as indicative of ADHD.

Defining Trouble: ADHD's Connection to Academic and Social Struggle

According to the APA, the diagnostic criteria for ADHD (see chapter 3) may be met after comparing a particular child's behavior to the perceived majority of children within the same age group. With regard to the plethora of ADHD symptoms, the APA claims that they must "have persisted for at least six months to a degree that is maladaptive and inconsistent with developmental level" (83-4). Such a "developmental" perspective is necessary because many of the behaviors that are supposedly linked to ADHD are typical of children in general. Therefore, a positive diagnosis of ADHD depends upon some kind of stark contrast between ADHD-suspected children and their peers. As their behavior is placed under rubrics of "maturational lag" and "slowed development," the discrepancy between ADHD children and their peers may be construed pathologically rather than idiosyncratically. As *DSM IV* does not categorically spell out a range of behaviors that are deemed to be "normal" for a given age category, the decision about what constitutes behaviors that are "inconsistent with developmental level" is highly subjective. On the basis of this analysis of parents' experiences with ADHD, I would argue that this subjective decision is largely contingent upon social dynamics that determine the difference between behaviors that are understood to be transitory and those that are believed to be indicative of something more fundamentally wrong with a child. Resonating with this diagnostic mode in modern clinical practice, parents describe the ways in which their children's ADHD manifested itself as academic and social struggle in school. As will be shown, parents make consistent comparisons between their children and others of the same age group with less difficulty in these areas.

Academic Failure

One of the most sociologically salient earmarks ADHD is its institutional specificity. In contrast to mental disorders that are reported to cause difficulty in a variety of social contexts (family life, romantic and work relationships, job performance, and so on), ADHD, as it is mainly detected in children, is a mental disorder whose point of discovery is almost inextricably linked to the institution of education. Corroborated by accounts from clinician participants, the troubles that most commonly spark the process of diagnosing a child with ADHD originate in the child's school. Such troubles are articulated in one of two ways: as academic struggles, denoting an inability to competently engage in the achievement of classroom assignments, and as social struggles, denoting interpersonal conflicts with other students and/or teachers. The former are often socially understood to be "personal" troubles, commonly involving initial remedial actions that are unofficial or informal, whereas the latter typify troubles that are relational, touching off remedial actions that are more technical and involve persons operating in official capacities (Emerson and Messinger 1977, 123). Both of these types of trouble adequately reflect the symptomatology of ADHD, namely that the disorder's inattention component can be seen in academic failure, and its hyperactivity component can be witnessed in children's overt behavioral problems. It is also important to note that the exhibition of these types of troubles may be aggregated in the so-called combined type of ADHD, in which academic and behavioral problems coexist (APA 1994, 85). Hence, with the symptoms of ADHD as decreed by the American Psychiatric Association, we see how "personal" and "relational" troubles may be conceptually synthesized into signs of the same mental disorder. As Emerson and Messinger (1977) describe, the definition of a specific form of deviance (in this case the designation of a child's having ADHD) is preceded by some understanding that troubles at one time perceived to be personal eventually become known as relational. This is illustrated by parents' accounts of their children's academic problems.

Both parents and teachers describe a lowering of academic performance as a point of concern prompting crystallized suspicions of ADHD. Such troubles are believed to become visible at a point in a child's school career when there is a discernible increase in academic demands—for most children diagnosed with ADHD, during or after their second-grade year. At their onset, these academic problems are often normalized, but when such problems persist and stand out among the child's peers, this normalization may be abandoned for more specific remedial efforts. Academic trouble becomes perceived as relational, not in an interpersonal sense, but as a general antagonism between a student and an institution perceived to be so crucial for his/her life chances. In the event that scholastic problems fail to be normalized through rationalization or general remedial efforts, social actors may assert a larger degree of formal authority and become more "official" in how they approach the child's struggles (Emerson and Messinger 1977, 121). These efforts may include conferences with parents, attempts to tutor, and intentional reductions in the expectation level of academic performance.

Parents who state that their children showed signs of academic failure most commonly describe difficulties in attention that are characteristic of the inattentive subtype of ADHD. Similar to the early observations made by Anna Freud (1926), parents commonly mention that their children exhibited "daydreamyness" and hence could not adequately participate in school lessons:

> Well, in second grade, we started noticing things with G. She was so daydreamy during class that her teacher approached us and told about some of her concerns. She had begun writing down some incidents and showed us what she was seeing. We had to start looking at her problem in a real way (stock broker, age thirty-nine).

Another parent discusses the same daydreamyness with his five-year-old son and mentions his son's self-diagnosis:

> At age two and a half he was into his own thing, not really paying attention outside of what was right in front of him. We thought, "OK, he's two." When he was about four and a half, teachers started paying notice to some of his problems. They kept telling us, "He's always daydreaming all the time." It's funny, I talked to him specifically about it. I asked him what was going on, why he wasn't able to focus. He said: "Dad, every time I start listening, my pants make a noise or I see something and when I get back to what the teacher is saying, I don't know where we are." Pretty good self-diagnosis for a five-year-old, eh? (schoolteacher, age thirty-seven).

It is commonly described that the condition of inattention emerges after children become older and consequently have more demands placed upon them. At the onset of these problems, adult figures, such as teachers, often normalize the tendency for young children (say between kindergarten age and second grade) to daydream, but this perspective yields to an intensified concern as the trouble perdures. In such cases, the scholastic incompetence of the child is no longer considered a stage of development but a solidified problem that is not going to "naturally" disappear. A thirteen-year-old eighth grader conveys a very similar experience: "For a pretty long time I was just able to get by. I think they all just thought I would be able to grow out of it, or like I would eventually get it and be up with the other kids. ...I think in second grade is when my mom and my teacher started becoming really concerned." A parent puts it this way:

> Well, when he was in first grade, we started noticing that he was having some problems focusing on the lessons. The teacher didn't think anything of it, but we were beginning to wonder if he was ever going to pass through this phase, which was what she called it. He also had big problems forming numbers and letters, even after most of the other kids started to get it down pretty well (graphic designer, age forty).

An emergence of the symptoms of inattention is a testament to the fact that many mental disorders are suspected after an individual's performance in an institutional setting is evaluated and deemed inadequate in relation to the performance of others. The term *phase* is imbued with normalcy, representing an expected collection of troubles that are believed to be rectified through a natural course of events. In its application, the word *phase* reveals how the summation of the essence of a trouble reflects the "intrinsic remedial measures" (Emerson and Messinger 1977, 126) used to rectify it—measures which, in the case of young children struggling in the formation of letters and numbers, may involve common, and nonalarming, pedagogical steps. When construed as a phase, daydreaming remains relatively unremarkable. As the trouble of daydreaming becomes noticeable in relation to the academic superiority of other children, it may engender mechanisms of more structured suspicion and assessment. Normalizing labels that are applied to daydreaming no longer have utility as the child's behavior is seen as indicative of a more paramount problem. It becomes difficult to assess scholastic incompetence as "a phase" as it is increasingly perceived to be abnormal in comparison to the performance of other students.

The mechanisms of troubleshooting that stem from consistent academic incompetence take many forms, assessments for ADHD and learning disabilities making up only a few types of evaluation. This is especially true in the case of older ADHD children. As one parent of a fourteen-year-old ADHD boy states:

> When he started failing out of school, we could really start to see that something might be really wrong. We knew it wasn't drugs or anything like that, but there was definitely something. His assignments weren't done on time and like every other day I was getting calls. The school psychologist...suggested that we run a blind drug test, which came back totally negative (housewife, age forty-two).

This trouble is addressed according to cultural notions of the kinds of problems adolescents may have. A possible case of drug abuse demonstrates a conventional way of troubleshooting academic failure in children who are considered older and susceptible to a larger array of social ills.

As academic failure is the primary "red flag" that prompts the suspicion of ADHD, it is not surprising that parents have much to say about their children's resentment toward the school environment. As one parent states: "He hates going to school. I have to unhinge him from my leg to get him out of the car sometimes. I don't know if that's ever going to stop" (property manager, age thirty-six). Such resistance commonly stems from the psychological struggles ADHD children have with academic requirements, social interactions, school disciplinary standards, and so on. Another parent mentions the psychological connection between school and failure: "He has decided that school is not the place for him. He associates school with failure. It's very frustrating for him" (postal worker, age forty-four). In accordance with psychodynamic discussions, ADHD is not necessarily seen through neurological impulses but through the psychological struggle children have with environments that demand prolonged task-oriented activity.

Parents convey that their children's resentment at school stems from a variety of sources, one of which concerns the way schools function as a labeling agent. As one parent explains, such labels for a child's troubles may be inaccurate:

> He really hates school right now. My husband and I are thinking about trying to get him into some other kind of program. The LAC work has not really worked because he thinks that we all think he is a dummy. And the administrators are starting to label him a bully, which is totally untrue (housewife, age forty-two).

Similar examples of resentments based in the social dynamics of schools and how these foster misdirected or embarrassing labels concern the way ADHD children are treated by their non-ADHD peers. One parent describes the failure of a "buddy system" that was established (and quickly discontinued) for the regulation of children's medication, and how this affected the identity of her eight-year-old son:

> For a while they tried a buddy system to help kids take their meds. The idea was that one kid would kind of watch out for the other and make sure that he took them. This was horrible for him because he felt embarrassed by the other children. All of the children knew he was taking meds. It got to where he wouldn't leave the car to go to school (legal secretary, age thirty-one).

Expressed here is the potential cruelty ADHD children experience when their condition becomes public knowledge. The child's resentment conveyed by this respondent resonates with teachers' statements examined previously claiming that the label of ADHD must be controlled and the normal identity of ADHD children preserved. In these cases the reaction to the ADHD condition and the pedagogical and treatment measures practiced by the school spark such children's resistance. Resentment is harbored as a result of schools, drawing attention to the disorder and compromising a child's normal identity.

Adding to the social variables that are perceived to affect ADHD children in schools are academic demands that are placed upon them. The bulk of parents describe their children as academically deficient, often conveying helplessness in facing the academic challenges presented by ADHD:

> Academically he is in the bottom 10 percent of his class. We have tried everything. Even with the medication it still isn't improving. He has been getting LAC time, and that seems to have some promise, but right now we just have no clue what to do (insurance underwriter, age forty-two).

Despite school interventions, including the efforts of special education teachers, school counselors, and school administrators, parents tend to express a degree of desperation about their ADHD children's academic prognosis and often attribute this to neurology: "In school he struggles a lot. His comprehension skills are also very poor compared to the other kids. That definitely led us to think it was a neurological problem" (dental assistant, age forty-one). Throughout the course of the interviews, discrepancies in performance between parents' ADHD children and their non-ADHD peers are repeatedly explained as a result of fundamental differences in neurology. Such themes reflect the dominance of neurological perspectives on ADHD.

Parents also describe the ADHD condition as becoming prevalent when scholastic environments changed. This is exemplified by a respondent who describes her child's experience in switching from a homeschooled environment to a public school:

> Well, my oldest was homeschooled up until his diagnosis. When he got into public school he was way ahead of the other kids. I worked with them both from 11 to 2 every day. I was in total denial because you couldn't really tell he had ADHD when he was being schooled at home. When he got into public school, he started at the top of the class and ended up at the very bottom. His teacher began calling every day because he started having serious disciplinary problems (legal secretary, age thirty-one).

For many parents, the visibility of ADHD symptoms is contingent upon environmental conditions. Intensive educational environments, such as those found in home schooling and in private schools with smaller class sizes, are argued to provide a psychological buffer and obscure ADHD from view. The public school environment, on the other hand, is argued to exacerbate the psychological frustrations associated with having ADHD and becomes the location where ADHD is more visible and more easily suspected. Parental denial, as indicated in the above excerpt, may become impossible to maintain as a child struggles in environments where the bulk of other children do not. As one boy, a ninth-grade student who was diagnosed with ADHD in third grade, states: "It was like I was stuck and I couldn't figure out how to get going again. …I think my mom didn't really know what to do or didn't want to see that I was having a real problem. …But after a while I was doing so bad there was nothing else to think."

The removal of denial is, I believe, part of a larger institutional commentary that stems from teachers' discussions of parental denial in the previous chapter. By repeatedly stating that they were "in denial" about their children's ADHD, parents presuppose that the ADHD condition was always there, but that their own psychological defenses obscured it from view. What requires further interrogation are the social dynamics of how denial is both realized and then broken. As its members do their best to build a case for ADHD prior to presenting such evidence to parents, the SBTeam is crucial in this regard. The process of building a case for ADHD is a way of removing parental defensiveness about the mental status of their children and is integral to organizing an increasingly sophisticated understanding of a trouble. As evidence is presented and soundly supported, it is argued, parents will have less room to offer rationalizations for their children's academic or social failings. In short, they will be less equipped to deny the allegations brought to them. Hence, when documenting discussions that repeatedly invoke denial, we must ask about the SBT's role in parents' description of this denial and also its role in parents' use of nomenclature that originates from SBT and other types of meetings with school representatives.

The discussions of other developmental conditions from which parents' ADHD children suffer demonstrate the relationship between parents and people who suspect and diagnose mental disorders. As one parent states:

> Well, he struggles a lot right now. He also has pretty severe
> dysgraphia. His short term memory is also very poor. We are
> going to have him tested for other LDs. Right now he is work-
> ing with the resource teacher, and I think he is making some
> improvement, but he just thinks that we all have him labeled
> as dumb or something like that (registered nurse, age forty-
> eight)

Parents frequently described themselves in an ongoing relationship with
one or more sources of mental health assessment. The label of dysgraphia—a fine-motor-skills disorder that distorts the way children draw
shapes and write letters—illustrates such previous assessments. This excerpt also exemplifies a parent's role in mediating between these forces
of diagnosis and their own child's identity. As described, a consultation
with the resource teacher is internalized as a sign that others think of the
child as "dumb" or incompetent.

Parents' accounts of their children's academic shortcomings often
highlight gaps in their children's learning. As one parent describes: "One
of the things his teacher has mentioned is that she thinks there may have
been some basic skills he missed in the previous grades. She says he is
reading on a third grade level. So, now, we are looking at getting him
some kind of learning assistance" (career counselor, age thirty-five).
Such children are not described as overall failures but are instead framed
as children who lack specific, attainable academic skills—a situation
quickly remedied given appropriate intervention. Other parents describe
specific shortcomings with their children, juxtaposing them with statements about skills their children wielded effectively:

> He has a pretty big deficit in his math skills and I would also
> say in his language skills. He wasn't reading until the end of
> second grade. But once he started picking it up, by now he is
> in the eightieth percentile. Once he gets something, he can run
> with it. But his oral skills are the most strong. His oral vocabu-
> lary is very impressive. People comment and say, 'I didn't
> know he knew words like that' (school teacher, age forty-
> three).

An account provided by a seventeen-year-old boy who was diagnosed
with ADHD at age ten corroborates this: "My thing was numbers. I just
couldn't get any of the math stuff. But when it came to reading, that was
my thing. I was always reading, in the car on the way to school, at lunch,

whenever." In addition to respondents who describe consistent academic failure, parents and children who highlight specific shortcomings in academic skills often describe areas of considerable academic competence.

The description of academic competence, or even of academic superiority, demonstrates a diversion from the neurological discussions of ADHD, which simply do not discuss areas in which ADHD children may have comparable or superior skills to their peers. The discussion of the more serious forms of ADHD are reputed to devastate the intellectual life of such diagnosed children, leaving little if any room for the discussion of other intellectual abilities. *DSM IV*, for example, contains no clause that states some ADHD kids may be prone to demonstrate an excellent vocabulary or may have better math skills than verbal skills. In drawing attention to academic strengths instead of weaknesses, parents and children reveal a belief in a uniqueness that transcends the generalizing tendencies of the ADHD label.

Furthering the discussion of academic competence and in opposition to the conventional wisdom claiming ADHD is characterized by academic struggle and the psychological association of school with failure, some parents state that their ADHD children are intellectually gifted and academically superior: "He's at the top of his class right now. He's ADHD gifted, which means that he has some pretty serious hyperactivity, but he is highly intelligent" (student, age thirty-three). The determining factors for ADHD in such cases strongly implicate behavioral troubles rather than strictly academic ones. Conflating mental disorder labels with those that denote intellectual prowess into the term "ADHD gifted" illustrates parents' nuanced way of understanding their children. This counters teachers' aforementioned assertions that ADHD children's academic problems and behavioral problems invariably feed into each other. From this perspective, parents frame their children as having an abundance of physical energy, and though they may have disciplinary problems, they also show intellectual strengths. The descriptions of these intellectual gifts are often coupled with discussions of ways that the school seeks to accommodate the special needs of these children:

> In fact, he is brighter than most of the other kids and performs very well, when given the right kind of direction. He has a real high IQ but was not able to regulate his behavior when he got into grade two. They put him in the APEX program for gifted children. ...They tried for a couple of weeks to make it work, but it just wasn't. With ADHD kids they're already bored eas-

ily, but being gifted on top of that kind of made him double-
bored (receptionist, age thirty-nine).

Certain children who are diagnosed with ADHD may not be overwhelmed by the demands of school but may actually be in need of extra
intellectual stimulation, according to some parents. In describing her son
as "double-bored," this respondent underlines the antagonistic relationship between ADHD children and school—a situation apparently exacerbated by the fact that her son is gifted. ADHD, in this regard, is framed
as a detriment to the implementation of advanced scholastic programs. It
is a disorder that thwarts the potential accomplishments of intelligent
children.

In drawing comparisons between the academic performance of parents' ADHD-diagnosed children and their non-ADHD peers it is curious
that ADHD kids are never once described as "normal" in relation to their
peers. ADHD children are either described as having some significant
shortcoming, or conversely, they are described as having some degree of
academic superiority to normal children. Being excluded from the normal category in academics highlights how ADHD is understood primarily through the requirements of the academic environment. This gives a
degree of credence to environmentally based arguments about ADHD in
which the disorder is argued to "exist" only under certain conditions. A
previous parent's discussion about her son's adjustment to public school
after excelling in a homeschool environment is a case in point. The perceived lack of academic normalcy in ADHD children may also be tainted
by parents' desire for their children to attain academic success. For example, an ADHD child may be performing adequately according to the
normal distribution in a particular classroom, but the desire to see children "be the best" may skew the way they are perceived.

Social Conflicts

Events that precipitate the suspicions of ADHD also include the exhibition of behavior that is considered directly antisocial, often violent. As
one parent states: "At age four he began getting violent. He'd take things
out of the bedroom and throw them into the hallway. One time he took
an air register out of the floor and threw it into a wall. We took him to a
psychologist after that" (postal worker, age forty-four). Such behaviors

are described as unprovoked and continued despite authority-figure intervention:

> Last year he was repeatedly aggressive and violent with the other children in kindergarten. He was also aggressive towards one of his teachers. She tried to pull him off a little girl and he acted like he was going to bite her. She says he was making some animal noises, but really scary and agitated, like he was totally out of control. None of this was happening during his preschool (student, age twenty-nine).

The defiance of authority figures is considered grounds for framing such violent behavior as abnormal and worthy of medical examination. Children who fail to cease violent behavior upon adult intervention are often labeled uncontrollable. As one parent states: "He got into a scrap on the school yard. He had this boy on the ground and he was putting the boots to him. A teacher intervened and he attacked her. You know how kids usually are when an adult intervenes; they stop what they're doing. But he had no way of controlling himself" (registered nurse, age forty-eight). In the event that an adult intervenes, it is commonly argued that children defer to that authority figure. However, when violent actions are not quelled by adult intervention, they are grounds for deeper concern. The history of a fourteen-year-old girl, who was diagnosed with ADHD just prior to the time of this interview, mirrors the violent situations described by parents. On an extended suspension from school for fighting at the time we spoke, this ninth grade student had and numerous clashes with her peers, also with teachers and administrators who tried to intervene. As she states: "I don't take no crap from no one. Not the teachers, no one."

The theme of violent behavior resonates with the clinical description of ADHD children who are believed to have a strong hyperactivity component to their condition, though most psychiatric positions would probably interpret such behavior as more akin to conduct disorder or oppositional defiant disorder. The interpretation of violent behavior as pathological seems more likely than in instances of behavior that demonstrates academic struggle. This has to do largely with the perceived gravity of violence and its social impact. Perhaps because violent behavior is seen as a threat to others and is blatantly disruptive, it is rarely conceived of as a phase. Almost any degree of violence, if apparently unprovoked, is considered to be grounds for concern. This concern is intensified when the remedial measures to thwart violent behavior (i.e., through the inter-

vention of adults) prove inadequate. The remarks of parents that address
the inefficacy of adults in stopping children from being violent, and also
their depictions of adults being attacked by such children when interven-
ing, describe the failure of remedial action and presuppose a more pathological condition with the child. The assumption of mental defect occurs
when the symbolic authority of adults has no effect. When adult authority is not recognized, it is assumed that the violent child must have a fundamental error in the way he/she internalizes symbols. Understood sociologically, the interpretation of childhood defiance as symptomatic of
mental disorder may also be a result of unrecognized adult power. This
epitomizes the "micropolitics" that Emerson and Messinger (1977) describe. In the case of child violence, the connections between such behavior and mental disorder stem from situations in which children do not
recognize adult authority. The power struggle between adults and children, from this perspective, is one that is rectified through formal evaluation measures.

Incidents that precipitate suspicions of ADHD also include acts of
self-directed violence. As one parent states: "I remember his first-grade
teacher mentioning that she caught him pressing a piece of glass into his
own hand. Not enough to break the skin, but it just didn't seem normal"
(receptionist, age thirty-nine). Another parent describes her six-year-old
daughter's attempt at hanging herself:

> Three years ago when my husband and I split up, it was really
> hard for my youngest. I guess to make up for the loss of their
> dad I decided it would be a good idea to buy the girls new kit-
> tens. My youngest went to tie a bow on the new kitten, and
> tied it way too tight. Well, I found the kitten which was totally
> unconscious and my daughter walked in and saw me trying to
> revive it. She thought she had killed it. She ran into her room
> and tied a skipping rope around her neck and tried to hang
> herself. After that I said, 'Well, you had better have both of
> these kids checked out.' I made an appointment with a psy-
> chiatrist and she said that both kids had ADD and that my
> youngest had ADHD (flight attendant, age forty-nine).

It is curious that such self-destructive behavior may lead to an ADHD
diagnosis instead of other mental disorders. Nowhere in *DSM IV* criteria
does it discuss a tendency for ADHD children to inflict harm upon themselves. A relevant question at this point is, How do acts of violence
against oneself and others constitute symptoms of ADHD? One answer

to this question may be found in the psychodynamic discussion of ADHD symptoms that describe problem behavior as a response to the consistent frustration that ADHD children encounter in everyday life. From this perspective, there is a seemingly endless list of behaviors that can be exhibited. To borrow from Emerson and Messinger (1977), the perceived severity of these behaviors determines the intensity of remedial action and whether or not the behavior itself is framed as symptomatic. Violent behavior, for example, may be rationalized as a coping mechanism on behalf of ADHD children to retaliate against a world they perceive as unyielding and hostile. Such behavior presumably points to a more fundamental condition.

Jason (pseudonym), a twelve-year-old boy I interviewed, had a social life that is considered typical of kids diagnosed with ADHD. Prior to being diagnosed at age eight, Jason began having marked academic and social struggles in school. As his inferior performance in school was becoming public knowledge to his peers, Jason became the brunt of abuse by other kids. He found himself often getting into fights and eventually became a regular in the principal's office. His social struggles in school extended into his life after school, in which he was rarely invited over to other kids' homes, and on the occasion when he would have a friend come over (invariably a child who was considerably younger than Jason), it always ended in some kind of conflict, either as a physical altercation or as hurt feelings. According to his mother, Jason overcompensated for his label in school as a "slow" kid by being overbearing with the few friends that he did have, and this always drove Jason further into isolation. Upon being diagnosed, Jason was immediately placed on Ritalin (10 mgs, twice per day), but severe adverse reactions, and the medication's failure to engender any change in Jason's academic and social situation, prompted his mother to cease the medication.[2] In seventh grade, at the time of this interview, Jason spends much of his academic time in special education and spends his leisure time largely alone or with his family.

Jason's story is typical because it describes how the perceived effects of ADHD can manifest themselves in a diminished capacity to make meaningful social connections. As repeatedly described by parents, these connections are largely taken for granted by other "more mature" children. The comparisons between ADHD children and their non-ADHD peers commonly depict ADHD children as "less mature" or not as sophisticated in social situations as one would expect from normal children of the same age. As one parent of a third-grade ADHD boy states: "Socially he is very far behind the other kids. His teacher was saying that his behavior reminds her of a first grader" (postal worker, age forty-four). The framing of social maturity in relation to others from the same age group is demonstrated through descriptions of the relative age of their ADHD children's friendship networks: "He has much lower social skills. All of his friends are much younger. I think it's because he's intimidated by older kids, or kids his age. He is very immature for his age" (nursing student, age thirty-eight). Other parents who mention discrepancies between their ADHD children's age and the age of their friends also add that their ADHD children struggle in the maintenance of friendships. As a parent of a twelve-year-old ADHD boy states: "As with other kids with ADHD, he is very socially immature. He has probably a ten- or eleven-year-old maturity. I think he has some problem making friends his own age and keeping those friendships" (registered nurse, age forty-eight). And another parent: "Socially you can tell he is not up with the other children. He isn't able to maintain friendships yet" (occupational therapist, age forty-two).

In cases like Jason's, in which physical altercations seem abnormally frequent, many parents claim that their children are prone to aggressive behavior around other kids and that these acts of aggression behavior precipitate ADHD diagnoses: "He has some difficulty with aggression and frustration, you know, lashing out at other kids sometimes. That's when he was diagnosed" (receptionist, age thirty-nine). Other parents give specific accounts of violence: "He is highly agitated, very aggressive towards others kids. He has bitten one kid on the nose already this year. That was the big call that he needed to get some kind of evaluation" (student, age twenty-nine).

In some instances parents say that their children's aggressive behavior also prompts mental health professionals to surmise the existence of other conditions. Describing her six-year-old son, the parent of two ADHD boys states: "He is a mixed bag according to the psychiatrist. He thinks there is a good chance that he also has conduct disorder. He is also really smart and manipulative, which is a symptom of ADHD" (legal secretary, age thirty-one). Such accounts of ADHD and aggressive behavior frame ADHD as comorbid with more blatantly antisocial mental disorders. Conduct disorder—a diagnosis rarely provided to six-year-olds—describes a tendency of children (usually boys) to feel compelled to act in aggressive and often violent ways. In addition to discussing the possibility that her son may be exhibiting signs of conduct disorder, this respondent also provides an interesting frame for her son's ADHD, namely, that his manipulative tendency is also a *symptom* of the disorder. This position represents a significant departure from dominant clinical narrative about ADHD, which draws no connection between ADHD and the ability to manipulate others.

When the Teacher Calls

Parents' discussion of the disruption of school activities primarily describe moments in which children stand defiant in the face of a teacher's authority. As one parent states: "He shouted back at his teacher when she told him to come join the group and refused to participate until she took him aside and talked with him. He disrupted the whole class until he felt OK and was able to sit down" (career counselor, age thirty-five). Another incident reflects the futility of teacher intervention:

> Well, in grade three we had an incident which was pretty telling. It was after recess and he wouldn't come back to class. People from the school were almost chasing after him trying to get him to come back in. It started raining, and he still wouldn't come back in. It was almost like a psychotic episode. They had to call me down and so I came down there and took him home because he still refused to come back to the class. We knew that something was pushing him to behave in such a way (housewife, age forty).

Similar to previous interview excerpts, this shows that the child's resistance to the wishes of authority are framed as "outside his/her own will." Such an incident is "telling" from this mother's perspective because it shows how her child, who should have been submissive to adult control, apparently is unable to exercise self-restraint. As G.F. Still (1902) would have said, this inability to submit to the wishes of adults may represent a "morbid condition," that is, the inability for self-control is understood to be embedded in the actual physiology of the child. Such conclusions presuppose that children, by nature, do not want to have the negative experience of being reprimanded or punished by adults. If they have a normal psychological development, it is assumed, they should understand the ramifications of their actions and be able to reflect upon their own behavior. In the event that an adult may not be able to control a child, assumptions may be made about the child's mental health.

The dominance of school as the primary location where "ADHD suspicious" incidents occur further demonstrates the significance of school as the major location for the detection of ADHD. The accounts from parents and children solidify the argument that suspicion of ADHD is directly related to antagonism between students and the institution of education. Because of this, we must interrogate the peculiar qualities of ADHD and its institutional specificity. On one side of this interrogation, we may state that the ADHD diagnosis has major validity problems. Recalling one clinician's comments calling ADHD a "garbage can diagnosis," we can surmise that ADHD is largely a catch-all typology for behaviors that schools deem disruptive and undesirable. Certainly such a position would be sympathetic to social constructionist arguments about ADHD. However, we may also conclude that ADHD, like other childhood disorders, is much more likely to be detected within a school environment, in the same way that autism or learning disabilities surely are. Such a position would proclaim that ADHD children do not find themselves in situations outside of school that are socially and intellectually complex enough to bring out the symptoms of the disorder. Once the classroom places intense demands upon ADHD children, the argument continues, their disabilities become visible. A psychodynamic perspective appears to serve as the rationale for parents in explaining that their child's ADHD behaviors seem to occur only during schooltime. Parents commonly mention that their child's ADHD-like behaviors only occur in the school context and justify this by claiming the school was a unique and more challenging intellectual and social context than, say, playing with the neighborhood kids or lounging in front of the TV.

I will state that with all of the children I was granted permission to speak with, all seemed very calm and comfortable in the surroundings of their home. One ten-year-old ADHD boy I spoke with lounged on the couch while watching television and seemed totally relaxed. It was difficult for me to think that this was a kid getting into constant trouble at school. When asked whether or not he liked school, he lazily states: "It's OK," then later includes that he felt school is "kind of boring sometimes." An eleven-year-old boy, and an avid Sony Playstation fan, claims that all of his problems are associated with school and that he generally cannot wait to get home, where it is, in his words, "more relaxing." As he states: "You don't really get to do what you want in school, I mean I don't know, the stuff we do is just not what I want to do." Such statements may be interpreted widely. On one hand we may claim that this boy's dislike of school is an extension of his own psychological problems, but on the other hand, the notion must be entertained that the school itself does not provide the avenues for learning that draw in certain types of children.

Many parents describe their children as quite normal outside of school. The apparent presence of ADHD is often attributed to the increased intellectual demands of that environment. As one parent states:

> When she's home she seems like she's doing quite well. She has her friends over and they play. Just normal kid stuff. I guess we really wouldn't even think she had ADD except for the problems at school. But if you think about it, it makes sense. The school is a place where greater demands are placed on the kids intellectually (stock broker, age thirty-nine).

Another parent emphasizes the social pressures that are inherent in the school environment: "At home he's very easy to be with. Loves to talk—he's a great talker—loves to visit. He's quite pleasant when he doesn't have all of the social pressure around him" (student, age thirty-three). Finally, another parent makes statements that resonate well with the issue of ADHD behavior and the resistance to authority: "I'd say the bulk of his problems have been in the school and are really between himself and the teachers. It's like these kinds of kids have a real problem with authority" (career counselor, age thirty-five).

Parents often report that when they are approached by parties from their child's school, those parties often express prior experience with the disorder. As one parent responds: "They said there was another boy who had been diagnosed with ADHD and they saw a huge difference when he started taking Ritalin. They also brought in a school counselor, and we got a referral to our family physician" (legal secretary, age thirty-one). Such statements refer to the end product of the SBT meeting and the compilation of information about a child before parents are contacted. A clinical referral, which is commonly prompted by the SBT, is a mark of the legitimacy of that group's recommendations. If their case is presented effectively, parents may act in ways that fit with school interests: recommendations for clinical referrals are accepted, children become clinically evaluated, and medication is often administered. Framed as entirely relational, that is, as antagonistic to others and ultimately damaging to the ADHD-suspected child, the child's trouble becomes urgent: "something must be done" at this point, and the mobilization of members of the SBT is a type of official action. These actions mark the beginning of "extrinsic remedies" (Emerson and Messinger 1977, 126), in which the interactions between troubled parties (e.g., ADHD-suspected students, their peers, their teachers, their parents, and so on) become mediated by individuals operating in a more official capacity.

As the interviews from clinicians demonstrate, school representatives are viewed as the most common group to approach doctors about a case of possible ADHD and the possibility of prescribing Ritalin. According to clinicians, parents approach clinicians after being prompted to do so by the school. Hence, parents often say that their opinions of their child's condition resonate with those of the school: "His first grade teacher suggested it (the possibility of ADHD). I was very inclined to agree with her, given his recent behavior" (student, age twenty-nine). In approaching clinicians, parents are representatives of school interest, and school interest is rooted in a strong desire to rectify problem behavior. The perceived ADHD know-how of teachers is integral in moving a child down the path to getting the ADHD diagnosis as long as parents comply with their recommendations. Such recommendations stem from teachers' professed academic knowledge of the disorder but are perhaps more effective when backed by considerable "everyday experience" with ADHD. By presenting themselves as people with experience in teaching ADHD students, teachers provide legitimacy to their authority in the detection of the disorder. As mentioned, their semiformal suspicion of ADHD children is highly effective in soliciting formal diagnoses. This is especially true for teachers experienced in special-needs children, particularly special education teachers: "I guess the first mention of ADHD was from his teacher. She had had some experience working as a special ed teacher and said that he probably had some kind of problem that couldn't just be ignored" (insurance underwriter, age forty-two).

Emerson and Messinger's (1977) assertions about changes in the perception of a relational trouble presuppose that the social acknowledgement of "something wrong" with an academically troubled student prompts the introduction of new people who serve in an intensified, "official" capacity. Though it is important to assert that official parties may become involved as initial efforts fail to remediate a trouble, this chapter highlights that the same individuals who apply remedial efforts can change their posture toward the trouble and adopt a more "official" stance on their own. Rather than simply deferring to those with ordained expertise, persons who take initial remedial action may draw upon their own expertise as a resource in further remedial efforts. The appropriation of the knowledge that comprises this official stance is indicative of a shift in social roles (e.g., the shift from teacher to "suspector") and may be as important in socially constructing mental disorder as the entrance of official parties who are considered as such through professional decree.

An indispensable framework for articulating the appeal to official authorities, or experts, to define and solve a trouble, Emerson and Messinger's (1977) essay draws necessary distinctions between the worlds of informal and official suspicion. Such a bifurcation may be further elaborated by analyzing how parties negotiate the boundaries that demarcate informal and official postures toward a trouble. The lay world is argued to try intrinsic remedial measures, perhaps tapping into its own interpersonal resources, and then, when the remediation fails, the trouble is shown to "outside parties" (Emerson and Messinger 1977, 121) involving a "circuit of troubleshooters," each with growing levels of sophistication (Emerson and Messinger 1977, 127). The term *outside* is explained by the authors as those parties operating in an impersonal official capacity, reconstituting the trouble as a "distinctly public phenomenon" (Emerson and Messinger 1977, 128). The interviews presented here further this definition by demonstrating that parties with personal connections to the troubled individual may also adopt a stance that is outside the immediate relational circumstances of a trouble. Teachers, for example, may be directly involved with a relational trouble concerning a student, hence having a personal connection to the trouble, but may also adopt an outside, official stance in response to this trouble. This is perhaps most clearly indicated when children's troubles appear to be directly antagonistic toward teacher authority.

The diagnostic and pedagogical functions of school, hybridized into a semiofficial form, demonstrate that suspicion may occur along a continuum rather than in a dichotomous relationship to the troubled individual and that points along this continuum can be adopted by a single person simultaneously. It is important to not interpret the semiofficial role of schools as indicative of collusive forces that have a collective interest in "inventing" ADHD. On the contrary, the previous assertions by some clinicians that teachers may be inappropriately practicing medicine demonstrate that even among agents who work with each other in addressing the same trouble, there remain struggles over the constitution of professional boundaries. The social transformation of a trouble into a case of ADHD illustrates the legitimation of official agents and their territories of knowledge and practice. As the social organization of a trouble unfolds, parents own the burden of tremendous social pressure. At one end, they must do what is necessary to keep their children involved with school, and at the other, they must negotiate the risks of diagnosing and treating their children. While it is clear that the conversion of a trouble into a medical problem is complex, once a "mental disorder" discussion begins, parents and their children are placed on a path in which their agency in interpreting the trouble is greatly reduced.

Notes

1. This chapter also devotes some space to children; however, due to the child respondent group being relatively small, excerpts from children's interviews should not be regarded as an in-depth analysis of children's experiences. Children's excerpts are brought in only to further illuminate themes that are pertinent to parents' experiences with their ADHD children.

2. According to his mother, Jason's reactions to Ritalin were so severe that she is now "turned off" by them and would not try alternative medications despite the pleas from their family doctor. Now twelve, Jason has been off medication for three years.

Chapter Eight

Developing Informal Expertise: How Parents Negotiate the Meaning of ADHD

As sociological and anthropological discussions of mental disorder depict, mental disorders, such as ADHD, become a shaping force in the life of the diagnosed person. This is the case for ADHD-diagnosed children and also their caregivers. Through the eyes of their educators, clinicians, and parents, the ADHD child's world requires regulation to promote the "management" of his/her disorder. Invariably, the active agents in this management are the authority figures surrounding ADHD children. In applying the ADHD mental disorder label, adults take on the responsibility for structuring a child's life to meet the perceived treatment requirements in conjunction with the diagnosis.

It is a matter of course that the most significant adults in the management of ADHD are parents. As we have seen in the previous chapter, parents are the primary mediators between their children and the agents of ADHD suspicion, diagnosis, and treatment; form relationships with persons owning considerable ADHD expertise; and are largely on the depraved end of an asymmetrical distribution of ADHD knowledge. The interactions between parents and ADHD experts demonstrate the role experts play in helping to define social problems (Brewer 1971; Meyer 1968). As the present chapter demonstrates, this asymmetry in knowledge is often greatly reduced as parents seek their own sources of knowledge about ADHD and apply the litany of clinical and popular perspectives on ADHD in their households and to their children. The "management" of the domestic environment, in this sense, is not the result of parental compliance with ADHD experts but is rather a result of parents filtering the vast amount of information about ADHD and applying it in ways that they find appropriate.

The Experiences of Finding Out:
Receiving Medical Validation

Within Emerson and Messinger's (1977) micro-politics of trouble framework, medically defining a problem can provide a sensation of relief: the parties who had been so frustrated by their failing remedial measures experience success in bringing the trouble to the attention of experts who categorically define it and prescribe its remedy. Hence, in discussing the point at which their children's problems became explained as a result of ADHD, parents' testimonies commonly illustrate the following experience:

> I was absolutely relieved to finally have someone define what his problem really was. I had known a little about ADHD prior to his diagnosis, so for me it wasn't hopeless and I felt that if we started dealing with it in time, we could make a difference (postal worker, age forty-four).

At the point of medical definition, the troubles that were previously indefinable and increasingly frustrating become clear and understandable. A seventeen-year-old boy expresses similar relief in reflecting upon when he was first diagnosed:

> I was a lot younger when the doctor diagnosed the problem, but I knew that something wasn't right with me. It was a relief to finally have someone else, you know, confirm that I was definitely not like all the other kids. It was like people had found out the truth. . . . I remember having a lot of hope that I was going to get more help with everything.

Feelings of relief reflect the fatigue associated with the social conflicts that accompany an unyielding trouble. Parents articulate that they had had suspicions of their children, that something was amiss with them, but failing an expert perspective, these suspicions remained unsubstantiated. For many parents, the moment ADHD was declared to be the root of the trouble validated their suspicions. As one parent states, finding out her son had ADHD was a moment in which she felt people were "finally listening": "I was relieved that someone was finally listening to me. I was trying to convince people for so long. It made sense that finally something was going to be done about this" (nursing student, age thirty-eight).

The first moments of "medical validation" bring knowledge that the ADHD trouble will be rectified, but this may also be combined with emotional experiences of shock, if not devastation. In the case of one 12-year-old boy I interviewed, his ADHD diagnosis was followed by a period of reclusive behavior; he spent the greater part of a week in the confines of his bedroom. According to his parents, such self-induced isolation was a way of coping with the shame associated with the ADHD label. In contrast to parents who immediately received the diagnosis as a step in a positive, treatment-oriented direction, such parents convey negative experiences, such as self-blame:

> I was truly devastated when our doctor said that he probably had ADHD. He referred us to someone who knew more about ADHD, but we all knew what was up. I did not know what to do. I blamed myself very harshly for his problems. Where I come from, a parent is responsible for all her child's problems. I was lost (insurance underwriter, age forty-two).

Such sentiment resonates with psychodynamic views that implicate family dynamics in shaping a child's behavior. If a child has consistent problems, especially in crucial institutions such as school, such perspectives blame larger family issues. This position is exemplified previously by clinicians who claim that ADHD is a collection of "little T" traumas throughout a child's life. The basis for many such traumas, it is argued, invariably rests with parents' relationships to their children.

Resistance and Acquiescence

There is a commonsense notion that children raised in "normal" households will extend this normalcy to their greater social relationships. Representing this perspective, some parents argue that their child's behavior, however troubling, was simply a representation of age or a common phase of youth that would pass as other troubles naturally do. School problems, for example, were perceived by some parents to be normal for most children and therefore not representative of ADHD: "I was shocked that her problems in school were being considered a mental problem. I always thought that most kids have some problems in school, but I never suspected it was something like this" (stock broker, age thirty-nine).

Normalizing perspectives on one's child exacerbates the sense of shock: troubles that were to be perceived as normal are now being framed by ADHD experts as pathological. Through their legitimacy as the definers of the ADHD phenomenon, the experts surrounding a case of ADHD mandate that parents adopt a disability perspective of their children. This adjustment in perspective reflects considerable expert influence, the experience of shock denoting a turning point in the way a child is perceived. One parent describes his experiences:

> Well, we were pretty blown away when the teacher first approached us with this. We didn't know how to react to it. I don't feel like we were in denial or anything like that. We just thought he was an active kid, doing what kids do. It came as a pretty big shock. Now, of course it's different. We understand a lot more about it and we don't see it as all that bad. It's a very manageable condition as long as you take part in its treatment (police officer, age forty-three).

A retrospective stance is visible in this passage—one that depicts a shift in perspective and a "breaking out of denial." Shock gives way to a medical understanding. The statement "Now of course it's different," bespeaks a subscription to expert perspectives that were previously a point of resistance.

A pathologizing perspective on ADHD children is a dominant part of the discourse that is directed to a parenting audience. Russell Barkley (1995b), for example, encourages parents to keep a firm mental picture of the nature of their child's condition and admonishes parents to "keep a disability perspective" on their child's behavior (Barkley 1995b, 134). Within this perspective, Barkley contends that parents should maintain a psychological distance from the problems of their ADHD child and avoid personalizing them: "This is hard, so you may have to remind yourself of your child's disability each day, perhaps even several times a day, and especially when you are trying to deal with disruptive behavior" (Barkley 1995b, 134).

In adopting a disability perspective on their children, parents are reminded to "stay on top of" the behavior of their children. Reminder systems, for example, are often recommended to parents and are used in a variety of ways by the parents I interviewed. Barkley (1995b), for example, recommends that parents place smiley-face stickers around places in their home in which parents frequently find themselves. "Whenever you spot a sticker," Barkley states, "comment to your child on what you like that the child is doing at that very moment—even if it is just quietly watching television" (Barkley 1995b, 131). Consistency in verbal praise is supposed to award nondisruptive behavior and cultivate more of it. The recommendation of smiley-faces shows that behavior modification techniques are directed not only at children but at parents, who need to be trained to manage their child's disorder. Technological devices are also involved in the process of disciplining parents. For example, Barkley (1995b, 131) recommends that parents use the MotivAider device to prompt them to reward children for good behavior or "check in" with their ADHD children at regular intervals. Initially intended for classroom use, the MotivAider ($90.00 retail cost) is a pocket-size, battery operated device that can be set to provide a gentle vibration at determined intervals for the ADHD child and/or parent. As the *ADD Warehouse* on-line catalog advertises: "The MotivAider sees to it that a child receives enough of the right reminders to make a specific improvement in behavior."

These and/or other types of regulatory needs that accompany the ADHD diagnosis are seen as highly daunting by some parents. Hence, acquiescence to medical interpretations of their children's troubles involve mixed emotional experiences, often described as a combination of relief and fear. As one parent describes it: "I was both relieved and devastated at the same time....I was scared for him, that he was going to have to struggle to get through this" (student, age thirty-three). Being afraid for one's child is concomitant with the confirmation that the troubles are more significant than normal disruptions and that rectification of these troubles would demand protracted attention. Another parent states: "I guess there was also an amount of grief on my part because I knew that my child was going to have to struggle through this for the rest of his life" (receptionist, age thirty-nine). Resulting from the ADHD diagnosis, grief is expressed in response to the loss of a child's normal status— something some parents appear to experience vicariously.

The experience of grief is indicative of Erving Goffman's (1963) notion of a "courtesy stigma" (29), which may be adopted by someone close to the stigmatized, often in cases of family association. As Goffman argued, the social ramifications of a stigma can be a part of the experiences of everyday life for those who are associated with the stigmatized. Such a condition provides grounds for asserting why the stigmatized can become abandoned by, or have strained relations with those closest to them. In "feeling" a child's loss, parents express sensitivity to the social ramifications of ADHD. In addition to fearing the perceived physiological problems associated with ADHD, parents are included in the ways in which the ADHD status affects their family.

Parents' Acquisition of ADHD Knowledge

As parents discussed those first moments of "finding out" that their children had ADHD and were now to be considered mentally disordered, their stories revealed how the emotional experience of shock gives way to strategies for managing their children's difficulties. What I found to be particularly interesting were the ways parents acquired knowledge about ADHD and used this knowledge to, first, soften the emotional blow of the diagnosis and, second, cultivate their own vigilance in the face of ADHD.

Connecting Suspecting Parties to Initial ADHD Knowledge Acquisition

Some parents describe their initial interactions with suspecting parties, usually teachers, as the beginning of the journey into ADHD knowledge. Parents often left those interactions with basic summary information about ADHD. As one parent states: "We first started learning from the stuff that his teacher gave us. It was a pamphlet and I think she might have given us a *Time* magazine article, or something like that" (finish carpenter, age forty-four). In this instance, the party who first suggests ADHD begins the process of parents' own education about the disorder.

In other instances, acquiring knowledge about ADHD may begin in a clinical setting, often with informational discussions about the disorder and the necessity of treating it. One parent describes her experience with a behavioral modification program at a children's hospital:

> He was finally diagnosed at [names a hospital]. We started their "At Home" program and went through some pretty intensive behavior modification stuff. We were told to "understand the diagnosis and defy the prognosis." I remember them also telling us that 80 percent of these kids will have drug and alcohol problems if the ADHD goes untreated (occupational therapist, age forty-two).

And another parent: "Our doctor gave us a pretty good description of what ADHD is, and this fit very well with both of them. He told us, 'If it isn't ADHD, the Ritalin will make him more hyper'" (legal secretary, age thirty-one).

What is of interest is the way information is given through the conversation with the clinic. In one instance, a parent is given an aphorism to follow ("understand the diagnosis and defy the prognosis") and a fact ("eighty percent of these kids will have drug and alcohol problems if the ADHD goes untreated"); in the other case a parent is told that if ADHD was not the condition, the medication would not subdue the child. The transmission of these bits of information represent moments in which parents are subject to the authoritative voice of the clinic, and given digestible facts about ADHD. One instance demonstrates that parents may be given authoritative opinions regarding the prognosis of untreated ADHD, the other, information about the effects of stimulant medication. These and other types of information function to urge the administration of medication: in one case, the use of stimulants is reputed to have the paradoxical effect of preventing illicit drug use, and in the other case, Ritalin—a stimulant very similar to cocaine in molecular structure—is reported to paradoxically affect ADHD children differently (i.e., by calming them down) from "normal" children.

This dissemination of facts about ADHD and the paradoxes of medication illustrated in the interviews are far from idiosyncratic and represent the influence of historical and contemporary ADHD discourse. This began with Charles Bradley (1937), who found it curious that Benzedrine, a drug known to foster increased activity in adults, provided a subdued reaction in half of the thirty children to whom he administered the drug. As he stated: "It appears paradoxical that a drug known to be a stimulant should produce subdued behavior in half of the children" (Bradley 1937, 582). Overall, Bradley saw the subdued reaction in these children as promising for future study. He remarked that the EEGs of these "paradoxical cases" were generally abnormal and that Benzedrine might have affected these cases differently than those with normal EEGs. His tentative conclusion: a physical brain abnormality may very well be linked to the paradoxical effect of Benzedrine. This seminal discussion of the "paradoxical effect" of stimulants upon mentally disordered children continues to be something which pro-Ritalin researchers attempt to prove (Conners 1972; Barkley 1991) and anti-Ritalin researchers attempt to disprove (Breggin 1998; Nicholls 1999).

C. Keith Conners's work strongly exemplifies the pro-stimulant, neurological discussion of the paradoxical effect of such drugs on hyperactive children. His 1972 *Pediatrics* article, "Psychological Effects of Stimulant Drugs in Children with Minimal Brain Dysfunction," marks the first attempt in the neurological literature to demystify and redefine the paradoxical effect. As he states:

> A number of myths have grown up regarding the behavioral effects and use of stimulant medications with children. The first is that there is a type of child uniquely responsive to stimulant compounds, namely, the hyperkinetic child. The second is that the hyperkinetic child is any child who is sufficiently overactive to be considered a menace by adults. The third is that the stimulant medications act primarily to reduce motor activity in a paradoxical "sedative" fashion (702).

In addressing the second myth Conners is responding to criticism concerning the validity of the MBD diagnosis, namely, the position that children diagnosed with MBD are not truly ill but instead are an inconvenience for authority figures.[1] Relevant to the topic of stimulants' paradoxical effects are the first and third myths Conners mentions, both referring to perceived misunderstandings about the physiological effects of stimulants in the brain. Such myths are addressed in a summary of his study of seventy-five (seventy male, five female) MBD children who were prescribed stimulants for their cognitive and behavioral problems. Such variability was found in the subjects' response to the medication that Conners categorizes the behavioral responses of the children into seven different groupings. Within these categories are only a few examples of stimulants having the "sedative" effect. This tremendous variation in children's' responses to medication prompts Conners to conclude:

> Thus it is apparent that there is both physiological and psychological heterogeneity in this group of children. All children with this diagnosis do not respond in the same way to drug therapy, and the types of response appears to depend on the profile of abilities, and possibly an underlying physiological responsiveness in the cerebral cortex (708).

By refuting the notion that the hyperkinetic child is uniquely responsive to stimulant medications (myth number 1), and that these medications act as a sedative (myth number 3), Conners suggests that MBD may take on many different forms and therefore reveal varying reactions to stimulants. MBD may be characterized by hyperkinesis or cognitive problems or varying combinations of the two. Keeping in line with psychiatric "reverse engineering" reasoning that views the responses to medication as indicative of the pathology being treated, Conners's study draws the conclusion that MBD is a syndrome as varied as children's responses to its treatment. The hyperkinetic or overactive child, according to this reasoning, cannot uniquely respond to stimulants because hyperkinesis is not the only manifestation of MBD. There are other components; attention-related problems, for example. Therefore, the assertion that MBD children are "susceptible" to the effects of stimulants and that this effect is generally sedative, are unfounded.

Conners's assertions, however, do not mean to be a declaration that stimulant medication acts in entirely unpredictable ways. Rather, his conclusion that the responses to the drugs are highly variable is a way of opening larger research questions concerning the effects of stimulant medication and why they apparently alleviate the behaviors associated with MBD. This question is implied in Conners's discussion of the relationship between "an underlying physiological responsiveness in the cerebral cortex" and the various and sundry effects of stimulants. Conners ponders the presence of a more sophisticated biochemical process in the MBD condition—one that may provide grounds for reinterpreting the condition's etiology. Such musings bore fruit when later researchers in the ADHD field asserted that the disorder was caused not by an overactivation of the brain but instead an *under*activation (Barkley 1997). Hence, the issue of the paradox of ADHD was recast by researchers in the field. Stimulant medications, they contended, acted exactly as they were supposed to: they sped up brain activity in the frontal regions of the brain. The paradox that needed to be understood, such researchers argued, was that the distractibility and hyperactivity so characteristic of ADHD reflected brain activity that was not too fast, but too slow.

Conners's (1972) discussion is an attempt to disprove the myths surrounding MBD children and stimulant drugs, but it reveals much about the process of how data are framed and how this framing can be used to further a line of research. For example, in accounting for the tremendous variability in his subjects' response to medication, Conners gives credence to children's "profile of abilities." To translate this: the response to medication may depend upon a child's cognitive strengths and which parts of the brain he/she uses best. What is peculiar (if not ideological) about this type of framing is how it ignores—and simultaneously discounts—the notion that there may be flaws in the diagnostic criteria for MBD. According to the principles of psychopharmacology, mental disorders are supposed to become discernible through a patient's response to medication. It follows, then, that a large variability in the response to the medication would imply that either the medication works erratically and/or the diagnosis has validity problems. Neither Conners nor his pro-stimulant contemporaries address these concerns. Despite the fact that validity problems concerning ADHD have never been rectified, parents appear to be widely taught that paradoxical effects, if they exist at all, prove the existence of ADHD.

The Pursuit of Literature

Upon being convinced to some degree that their children had ADHD, parents describe a voracious appetite for information in the pursuit of ADHD knowledge. "I started reading everything I could get my hands on," one parent, a stock broker, age thirty-nine, tells me. Gaining ADHD knowledge is done with a sense of urgency that is prompted by the grim prognosis of untreated ADHD and parents' desires to bridge the gap in understanding their children. Knowledge and the hunger for it, in this sense, are tools of empathy. As one parent states: "I did whatever I could do to learn more about his condition and why he did the things he did" (Student, age twenty-nine). Through acquiring information about ADHD that would enable a deeper understanding of their children, most parents I interviewed had accumulated a great deal of ADHD resources, mostly in the form of printed matter. As one parent admits: "I have a library of information in my house; no joke, I must have thirty books on ADHD" (postal worker, age forty-four). Found in the homes of the parents I interviewed was a substantial cross-section of ADHD guide books. Some of the more popular of these include: Colleen Alexander Roberts's *ADHD and Teens* (1995), Russell Barkley's *Taking Charge of ADHD* (1995), Grad Flick's *Power Parenting for Children with ADD/ADHD* (1996), Edward Jacobs's *Fathering the ADHD Child* (1998), and Paul Weingartner's *ADHD Handbook for Families* (1999).

Though this cross-section by no means exhausts the available ADHD parental guidebooks, the contents of these and other texts are reflected in many of the ways parents view their ADHD children. Such guidebooks shape parents' perceptions and may be read as "ideological representations" (Smith 1990, 83-100), that provide templates for how the household needs to be restructured, or at least, rethought, to meet the special needs of ADHD children. ADHD guidebooks are based upon particular frames for ADHD, to the exclusion or dismissal of alternative opinions on the disorder. From Dorothy Smith's (1990) point of view, the text most read and most legitimated has won a kind of ideological battle. This ideology does not end at the point of the written word but manifests itself in the social practices of individuals, their behavior, and their everyday language.[2] Examining such literature provides insight into the textual side of the relationship between discursive formation and the lived experience of ADHD parents. Smith (1990) offers a description of this relationship:

> Such textual surfaces presuppose an organization of power as the concerting of people's activities and the uses of organization to enforce processes producing a version of the world that is peculiarly one-sided, that is known only from within the modes of ruling, and that defines the objects of its power (83-4).

The ADHD parental guidebook summarizes the "experience" of ADHD, that is, it tells the audience what ADHD is like and professes knowledge of the best way to treat the ADHD condition. ADHD is placed within a "mode of ruling," which determines the ways in which the disorder is to be understood and the appropriate methods for its treatment. Implicit within this literature is the assumption that ADHD children are "abnormal"and that measures must be taken to aid them in living a "normal" life. Hence, in conjunction with its conceptual schemes, the ADHD guidebook documents specific techniques of behavioral reform.[3]

The way such sources of information restructure parents' thinking about ADHD is seen multifariously in the interviews. For example, parents who had gained knowledge of ADHD from such resources appeared to have contentment through knowing the "truth" about the disorder. Consequently, I was implored by parents to understand the bases for their own conclusions about ADHD. One respondent insisted that before the interview I sit at her table and explore her considerable stack of academic and popular articles, pamphlets, books, and so on. Many parents describe that they had reaped the fruits of their labor in studying such material and gained considerable expertise about ADHD. As one parent states: "Now I feel like I'm almost an expert on the topic" (insurance underwriter, age forty-two). In many regards, such parents certainly are ADHD experts on par with the clinicians I interviewed, and in some cases the parents have superior knowledge to them.[4]

In expressing this expertise, parents convey allegiances to particular books on the ADHD topic. One parent gives an example: "I first learned about it from some print-offs on the internet and then I began the book buying. *Driven to Distraction* was the one that I really got into" (legal secretary, age thirty-one). The best selling ADHD guidebook in print, Edward M. Hallowell and John J. Ratey's *Driven to Distraction* (1994) is mentioned by numerous parents as a significant introduction to the topic of ADHD. *Driven* adopts a less stigmatizing stance towards ADHD, framing the disorder as a normal condition, a personality trait that has lost its place in our modern, limiting culture. Because of its normalizing approach to ADHD, the text strikes a rare balance between raising awareness of a mental condition and rejoicing in the uniqueness of people, reflecting many of the perspectives parents have of their ADHD children. The allegiances to texts such as *Driven* demonstrate how parents differ from teachers and clinicians in their motives for learning about ADHD. Unlike teachers and clinicians, who have professional goals in looking at the disorder on an objective, "case-by-case" basis, parents preserve a degree of mysticism about their children and eschew some of the all-encompassing arguments about the nature of an ADHD individual. *Driven* is an excellent appeasement to the desires of parents because it provides an account of ADHD—and certainly forms some generalizations about it—while avoiding an overriding character summary of each and every ADHD person.

Driven is also popular because it is a parent-oriented book in which the authors (both physicians) claim to have the ADHD condition. Because of the authors' autobiographical account of ADHD, this text, like the others previously listed, enjoys a tremendous credibility with its audience. The credibility of ADHD texts that are directed at parents is commonly established through this modality, also known in interpretive sociology as the "personal experience story" (Denzin 1989, 38). For example, in the *ADHD Handbook for Families*, Weingartner (1999, vii) begins by telling his readers that he is diagnosed with ADHD: "Well, I wasn't lazy or retarded or acting out to get attention. I had—and still have—attention-deficit/hyperactivity disorder," and he is now in the profession of helping people with the disorder. Next to the author's photograph, the back cover of Alexander-Roberts's *ADHD and Teens* (1995) states: "Colleen Alexander-Roberts is the mother of two children with ADHD." In conveying their experiences with ADHD, authors place themselves "in the know" in relation to their readers, occupying the same "team" as their interlocutors (Goffman 1959, 77-105).

Parents Theorizing the Nature of ADHD

Most of the aforementioned parent-oriented literature tends to frame the causes of ADHD in a variety of biological ways. *Driven to Distraction*, for example, explores the possibility that ADHD is an unspecified, genetic personality trait, while others explain ADHD in different biological terms. Given the breadth with which the parent-oriented literature uses biologically oriented arguments to substantiate the nature of ADHD, it is not surprising that parents have similar variance in their accounts of the causes of the disorder.

The Various and Sundry Uses of Biology

In articulating that ADHD is genetic, parents exonerate child-rearing styles and/or traumatic events for creating ADHD symptoms. Among the most common accounts parents give for the causes of their children's ADHD, genetically based arguments cast ADHD as inevitable, a condition that may show up in the DNA strand at any time. Appeals to such arguments place the genetic hypothesis against the backdrop of the greater society or against the backdrop of one's own family. In some instances parents look to the behavior of members of their own families, including themselves, to demonstrate the genetic nature of ADHD. In other instances, parents adopt a more "human species" approach, arguing that ADHD is a character trait of the greater gene pool.

Taking the anthropological, gene pool approach to ADHD, some parents claim that people who are today labeled with ADHD were actually some of the most useful members of earlier societies. ADHD, in this sense, is atavistic. As one respondent (herself diagnosed with ADHD) states, people with ADHD are the ones who have a difficult time being molded to the constraints of modern society:

> It's all part of the DNA. From the beginning of time we were the survivors. We are more nature people, not technical people. The society we have has placed us into some pretty rigid spots. We aren't really able to be who we are. So, they call it ADHD, but it is really a sign of a survivor (flight attendant, age forty-nine).

From this perspective, labeling a trouble "ADHD" is a function of history. The assumption is that during an earlier time people who would today be labeled ADHD were highly valued members of society. People with ADHD, such parents argue, are more sensually connected to their surroundings, constantly in tune with the stimuli around them. In a society where an emphasis is placed on repetitive and focused kinds of activity, such personality types are deemed unproductive and a nuisance.

Other genetic stances toward ADHD adopt a familial position. Parents responding in this manner often state that they could see ADHD in their families or in themselves. A brief response by one parent exemplifies this: "I think it is familial, genetic. When I look at my own family tree, my mother has it and I think I may have traces of it" (registered nurse, age forty-eight). As another parent demonstrates, the familial connection to ADHD may be made by opposing the characteristics of the two sides of the family:

> I do think it's genetic. I have wondered about myself, you know, whether or not I might have ADHD. I know that it doesn't come from his mom's side. They're all incredibly organized, high-achieving people. Who knows? I may have a touch of it. I was never a very good student either (police officer, age forty-three).

In further confirming a biological view towards ADHD, parents explain that their children's disruptive and punishable behavior could not have originated from willfulness but is instead attributable to a "non-human agent" (Weinberg 1997; see the previous chapter). ADHD children are said to be driven beyond their own notions of right and wrong. This stance follows the discussion of ADHD demonstrated in chapter seven which states that children, by nature, do not desire punishment. Hence, consistently being in trouble is considered symptomatic of a larger condition:

> I think it's definitely biological. There is no way [mentions son's name] would act like that intentionally. He is driven by something outside of his control. That's why he gets so frustrated with other people and has to lash out. Now, I don't know what causes this, but I can tell you that it's real (student, age thirty-three).

When acting out, children may be punished for behavior they cannot control in the first place. An unsavory cycle of behavior and punishment is believed to engulf ADHD children, whose self concepts are damaged and whose negative attitudes towards crucial institutions crystallize.

Many of the parents I interviewed continue the discussion of ADHD as a non-human agent by invoking various theories about ADHD as a type of brain malfunction. Such discussions lack the jargon-laden descriptions that some clinicians provide. No parents mention the frontal lobe or basal ganglia as a location of their children's ADHD. In addition, some accounts reflect the overall uncertainty concerning the causes of ADHD. Some discussions, for example, contain contradictory statements. The following excerpt serves as an example:

> Well, I definitely think it's a physical thing. The wiring is not firing all the way when they get into certain environments. Out on the playground or in the gym they do fine, but put them in a class or in front of a new teacher and they just go haywire. I think that kids are born with this, and some learn to cope, but there are some, like my kid, who just have too much brain activity, just too excitable in certain situations (postal worker, age fort-four).

The term *wiring* alludes to the physical makeup of the child's brain, and how it processes stimuli in different situations. A contradiction is clear in this excerpt as this parent likens ADHD to a condition in which "the wiring is not firing all the way" but then later states that ADHD may also be a result of "too much brain activity." The volatility of ADHD children is invoked, in which they may fail academically and/or have behavioral outbursts. The former case may denote having too little brain activity, whereas the latter may be linked to too much. Such responses demonstrate some of the contradictory ways ADHD is understood in both popular and clinical realms. Demonstrated previously, clinicians also have very divergent views about what causes ADHD, as some believe it is a result of brain inactivity, whereas others contend that ADHD may result from brain overactivation.

The relationship between abnormal brain activation and the presence of ADHD is repeatedly connected to the effectiveness of stimulant medications. In conveying certainty that the ADHD diagnosis is correct, such parents say that the effectiveness of stimulant medications bolstered their belief in the validity of the hypothesis that their children's problems stem from specific brain problems. One parent, for example, describes how her son's response to Dexedrine is sufficient evidence for the presence of ADHD:

> When he took Dexedrine it was clear that he was being treated for something. He said, 'Mom, it makes things less fuzzy.' The only thing is he didn't want to take it during hockey game days. So we said, 'OK, you don't have to take it then.' But his behavior was definitely different on the days when he wouldn't take the medication (housewife, age forty-two).

In addition to how such responses reflect psycho-pharmacological modalities in psychiatry, it is arguable that at the moment of the expert suggestion of ADHD, alternative perspectives on the nature of childhood misbehavior become less possible. Because it comprises so many different symptoms, the ADHD label can be applied in a variety of different ways. Recalling the *DSM IV* criteria for ADHD, symptoms that warrant suspicion of the disorder comprise both introverted and extroverted behaviors. Furthermore, these criteria become even more inclusive when examined outside of the confines of *DSM IV*: within classrooms and inside homes. As seen thus far, parents attribute self-mutilation, manipulation, and outbursts of violent behavior to ADHD. Therefore, being convinced that the initial ADHD diagnosis is the right one does not necessitate that parents understand the disorder uniformly or that every clinician address it similarly.

Parents also give reference to specific theories about ADHD but may do so in a tentative fashion. As one parent states:

> I am convinced that ADHD is a result of brain chemistry. There's just an imbalance in the brain somewhere. I heard that the neurons get interrupted, like they're unable to fire and completely finish a task. The brain isn't aroused as it should be—it's kind of sleeping (occupational therapist, age forty-two).

This parent then directs me to Gabor Mate's *Scattered Minds* (2000)—a text I had read at the time of the interview—as the location of his knowledge about the physical properties of ADHD. The unsure language at the beginning of this response—for example, stating that ADHD is caused by "just an imbalance somewhere"—gives way to the invocation of some specific theories about the disorder. In this instance, this parent directs me to Mate's position about brain underactivation and his "traffic" metaphor, which likens the brain of an ADHD child to a traffic intersection in which the mechanisms for directing traffic are asleep at the switch. The inactivity of brain regulation mechanisms causes chaos in the way the brain processes information. The different cars (metaphors for neurotransmitters) do not know when to stop or go. Children with ADHD are therefore said to be drawn in every direction, unable to filter important stimuli from the unimportant, and they become hyperactive. From Mate's perspective, this condition contributes to the paradoxical appearance of ADHD: less brain activity leads to seemingly hyperactive behaviors. Though *Scattered Minds* does not posit new research findings about the origins of ADHD, this bestselling text is relevant for understanding how ADHD children are perceived within the clinic and the household. The text is geared for a popular audience, its etiological positions on ADHD strongly mirroring dominant neurological perspectives on the disorder. The invocation of Mate and application of his ideas represent the filtration of research-based knowledge through popular texts into the knowledge base of parents.

Exploring Nonmedical Alternatives

Though there is a clear connection between biological understandings of their children's ADHD and the literature parents read, many of my conversations with parents reveal an ongoing process of negotiation between their children's welfare and the recommendations of ADHD experts. Both the parenting literature and some of the parents in my sample explore external influences on ADHD behavior, promoting the regulation of specific household activities. Of particular concern are eating, television viewing, and the playing of video games. With regard to ADHD and diet—a discussion started in the early 1970s—it is argued that ADHD symptoms are externally caused by the body's reaction to artificial food additives. Television and video gaming are also attributed a causal status in ADHD, but part of this discourse also argues that ADHD children are much more sensitive to these stimuli than other children, therefore requiring a special regulation of these behaviors.

The Feingold Diet

Many parents who sought alternative diagnoses and treatment for their children explored the linkage between their child's diet and misbehavior. For some parents, such an approach to ADHD was attempted, but considered to be too daunting: "When he was younger we looked into diet to see if it was affecting him, but that was a very tall order. After a couple of weeks, it just fell apart, long before we could see any positive results" (insurance underwriter, age forty-two). The difficulty of such dietary interventions into ADHD is exemplified by my visit with a twelve-year-old ADHD boy and his mother. As his mother and I talked I could not help but notice all of the processed "junk" foods that lay around the kitchen and the can of Coca Cola this child drank as he paced around the kitchen while his mother and I were doing the interview. I later remarked in my notes: *Isn't Coke loaded with caffeine, and wouldn't this affect hyperactivity?* Clearly, in a society where processed foods are the dietary norm, seeking alternative food sources can be highly problematic.

Another parent, whose methods included the elimination of artificial food additives, states: "We've tried a lot of diet stuff. My wife and I have read a lot of stuff about diet and it affecting behavior. A homeopathic doctor had us cut out red dyes and MSG. He also gave us some herbs to help with his sleeping. His insomnia got pretty bad when he was on the medication" (occupational therapist, age forty-two). Implied in this passage are some of the common side-effects of stimulant medications, specifically insomnia. In consulting homeopathic doctors or in seeking treatment remedies that fall outside the pharmaceutical mainstream, parents are exhibiting a genuine concern for the long-term health of their children. As in the case of more conventional (read: biological) interpretations for the children's problems, parents who seek alternative explanations reach out to established discussions in these areas. In the early 1970s, for example, clinical discussions linked hyperactivity to food additives.[5] The most influential of these positions is known as the "Feingold diet" (Feingold 1974), which required that parents rigorously document the presence or absence of such additives during times when their child acted undesirably.

In *Why Your Child Is Hyperactive* (1974), physician Ben Feingold systematically outlines why food additives are linked to hyperactivity. Approaching retirement before the barrage of medical discussions of hyperactivity during the late 1960s, Feingold wrote: "Suddenly, retirement did not interest me. I launched into educating myself on the problems surrounding the hyperkinetic child" (Feingold 1974, 17). As a pediatrician turned allergist, Feingold was very interested in seeking allergenic reasons for what the media had presented as an increasing learning and behavioral childhood deficiency. Feingold asserted that the problems of inattention and hyperactivity were a new phenomenon—something he had not seen in fifty years of pediatric practice: "I had no recollection of a high frequency of hyperactivity and behavioral problems through all these years" (Feingold 1974, 19).

For Feingold, the problems of hyperactivity were new to a culture that was increasingly using artificial means to enhance the taste and color of its food. In addition to providing a new theory about what caused hyperactivity, Feingold served as a cultural critic. His work acknowledged that consumers derive sustenance from foods with polysyllabic, artificial ingredients and hypothesized that these had unrecognized adverse effects. For Feingold, that cultural moment of artificial nutrition was most visible within the household, where adults fed their children. Feingold endeavored to raise awareness of the types of foods people consumed, and implemented practices to regulate their consumption. His assertions countered much of the neurological discussions of hyperactivity during that time. When biological theories about hyperactivity were becoming dominant, Feingold's work represented a growing skepticism about the organic causes of hyperactivity and its treatment with stimulant drugs. His book denounces the use of medications, citing case studies where he had children taken off medication and placed on an additive-free diet. Referring to the case of "Johnny B," Feingold states: "With absolutely no drug support, the next three weeks were very erratic, both in the classroom and on the playground. Schoolwork, however, continued to improve rapidly. The home behavior remained good. There was no reason to panic and place him back on drugs" (Feingold 1974, 38). Feingold became famous because he offered a nonmedicinal solution to a problem believed to be inextricably bonded to pharmacology since the first prescriptions for Ritalin were written in 1961. The responsibility for treating hyperactivity could be removed from drug-dispensing clinicians and placed into the hands of parents, who would have to keep a close eye on their children and watch what they ate and how they behaved. The results of this scrutiny, Feingold contended, would be worth their effort.

Feingold suspected that numerous food additives caused hyperactivity, but had particular concern with Food, Drug, and Cosmetic (FD&C) Yellow #5. A common additive in everything from breakfast cereal to children's vitamins, FD&C Yellow #5, or Tartrazine, Feingold argued, behaved "within the human in the same manner as a drug used for medication—a fact some physicians overlooked" (Feingold 1974, 6). Feingold argued that the presence of this additive and/or others was a consistent variable in over one hundred cases of hyperactivity he treated, and if a careful log of diet and behavior was maintained, the effectiveness of the new diet could be substantiated. Feingold gives an example of this type of documentation in the case of "Johnny A":

> The next day, a Saturday, Johnny A began rigid food and beverage management. His dedicated mother, a remarkable woman, began a diary that lasted, with few breaks, until April 16, 1973.
>
> ...On the 18th Johnny had spaghetti for dinner. The sauce was homemade. She wrote: "I goofed. Used Tomato sauce but there was no obvious behavior change.
>
> ...Tuesday, the 21st, she underlined chocolate bar. "At 11:30. Very noticeable behavior change by 2:30.
>
> *From that incident on, a pattern developed. Any candy infraction (store-bought), ingested singly, appeared to cause a reaction in two to three hours.*
>
> Wednesday. A question mark. "Something off diet here. Slight behavior change."
>
> *I checked the items. Perhaps the breakfast bacon was artificially flavored with hickory.*
>
> ...December 1: "1 teaspoon of antihistaminic cough syrup at bedtime produced a raving maniac the early part of December 2."
>
> *I knew the brand. It was both synthetically flavored and synthetically colored* (32-33).

This passage represents the relationship between the interests of a medical practitioner and a "remarkable" mother. At least two social roles are present: first, the role of mother as "dietary archivist," and second, Feingold as postulating physician. The mother documents what her son eats and how he behaves; the italicized words, obviously the contemplative voice of Feingold, are in direct response to her observations. The relationship between Feingold and Johnny A's mother reflects how the household can become a location for a rigid documentation of childhood behavior, and in so being becomes a proving ground for medicalized forms of discipline.

Television and Video Games

Parents also say that part of disciplining their ADHD children involves a somewhat strict regulation of television and video games. Upon receiving their child's diagnosis, some parents, for example, made watching television a "weekend only" activity that in the words of one parent was for "times when kids can be a little more distracted." In addressing this issue, parents also seem to sympathize with the notion that the images from television and video games exacerbate their children's ADHD symptoms. Similar to the discussion of diet and ADHD behavior, the discourse of ADHD symptoms and television and/or video games is also a significant part of the cultural commentary that addresses children's hyperactivity and inattention. This discussion adopts two significant themes: (1) that ADHD children are in need of special television regulation; and (2) that television is a causal factor in ADHD symptoms.

Grad Flick (1996) contends that television needs to be regulated in any home, however, television is one of many "Special Problems for the Child with ADD/ADHD" (Flick 1996, 105-123) requiring particular regulation in such cases. He states: "Compared with movies, TV is also regulated much less by the parents. In fact, many parents may be surprised to hear what type of TV shows their child may watch when not supervised. What can you do?" (Flick 1996, 115). The ADHD child, Flick asserts, is especially susceptible to violent and aggressive television images. Such television programming "makes it more difficult to deal with children's social behavior problems, and especially those of the child with ADD" (Flick 1996, 115). Barkley (1995b) expresses a similar view: "While exposure to the violence that seems endemic in so many children's programs, including cartoons, usually doesn't increase the aggressiveness of normal children, it can do so for children already prone to aggressive and impulsive behavior, such as your ADHD child" (Barkley 1995b, 184).

In *The Myth of the ADD Child* (1995)—a text written to debunk many of the neurological conceptions of ADHD—Thomas Armstrong asserts that television could be one of the reasons childhood behavior has begun to deteriorate: "in the case of certain Nintendo-crazed, television-addicted youngsters, broader cultural issues could become primary" (Armstrong 1995, 34). Armstrong's text, devoted to providing "50 ways to improve childhood behavior without drugs," lists television regulation as an important aspect of controlling child behavior. On his list of fifty, television regulation is number three (Armstrong 1995, 75-78). He recommends that parents drastically limit the amount of television a child watches and totally eliminate violent programming of any kind in their household.

Richard DeGrandpre's *Ritalin Nation* (1999) expresses similar sentiments about the effects of television. DeGrandpre's argument is entirely devoted to describing ADHD and the rampant use of Ritalin as strictly cultural phenomena, having no basis in clinical reality. His analysis implicates the social effects of television on youth:

> That so many people drift into TV world without thinking, or find that they cannot separate from it once it's on, tells us how easy it is to forfeit self-control and succumb to the never-ending providers of effortless stimulation. In the case of children, this takes its greatest toll, for we know that they are much less likely to develop other ways of occupying themselves—other habits, other skills—as long as the television sits on its throne, staring down at them (25-26).

DeGrandpre insists that ADHD symptoms are the result of an over-stimulated populace, that falters when presented with challenges of the everyday world. These "other habits, other skills," so crucial to normal functioning, are nonexistent in a culture DeGrandpre claims is plagued by television and a litany of other "sensory addictions" (DeGrandpre 1999, 31).

Armstrong and DeGrandpre's TV etiology, much like Ben Feingold's dietary etiology, stand strongly opposed to neurological positions towards ADHD. Similar to Feingold, both Armstrong and DeGrandpre examine hyperactivity from a cultural rather than biological perspective. A culture inundated with fast-moving images and constant visual stimulation mirrors the thoughts and behavior of its children. The psychologically harmful forms of culture are not going to disappear, Armstrong and DeGrandpre imply. Instead of subscribing to a neurological myth, and, in effect, "blaming the victim" in the case of ADHD, both authors suggest that the domestic sphere should exercise more control over the interaction between child and culture.

Suspicions of television being a causal ADHD variable have owned a small, yet not insignificant, part of psychiatric discourse. For example, in a letter to the *American Journal of Psychiatry*, Matthew Dumont (1976) states:

> I would like to suggest that the constant shifting of frames in television shows is related to the hyperkinetic syndrome. Television has emerged as the single major cognitive experience during the developmental years of huge numbers of children. Apart from the vapid and violent content of the programs, there are incessant changes of camera and focus, so that the viewer's reference point shifts every few seconds. This technique literally programs a short attention span and probably accounts for the almost hypnotic attraction television has for many of us (457).

Dumont goes on to argue that it is problematic for children to be expected to behave in the classroom when their television-influenced frame of reference has no isomorphism to the dullness of classroom structure. In addition, Dumont hypothesizes that "amphetamines control this behavior by providing a subjective experience comparable to the fleeting worlds of television and hyperkinesis" (Dumont 1976, 457). Dumont's letter also expresses a cultural etiology. The administration of medication might not be linked to the regulation of a neurological imbalance as much as its effect might mimic a type of world that children have become accustomed to, if not hypnotized by. Medication calms children because it makes the world appear familiarly hyperreal.

Authors who associate television with hyperactivity and inattention argue that the fractured experience of television, in that it is a normal part of childhood, is something that children carry with them into a variety of institutional settings. A crucial institution in this regard is education. In *Go Watch TV!* (1974, 164) Nat Rutstein states: "Too many children sit in classrooms in body only, thinking technicolor thoughts of distant lands and beyond, where Star Trek circulates, of the moon, where astronauts pick for clues, and of being back home, embraced by television beams." A similar stance is taken by Marie Winn in *The Plug-in Drug* (1985) in which she argues that children's educational shows, such as *Sesame Street*, make children equate learning to a technicolor, scene-shifting experience. The classroom, in comparison, is a boring letdown, responded to with restlessness and contempt. This sentiment is also expressed in a more recent study of video games by Steve Dorman (1997), which contends that "a more subtle impact of video game technology on education is the expectation by children that all learning must take a gaming approach and be fun" (Dorman 1997, 136; for other examples of literature that explore the relationship between video games and childhood behavioral problems see Bruno 1995; Keepers 1990; Soper and Miller 1983).

The fairly extensive clinical and popular discussion connecting television and video games to child hyperactivity and/or inattention is as much a commentary on the nature of domesticity as it is one about contemporary media. The world view that is inculcated in the image-saturated living room, numerous authors assert, has a lack of fit with the outside world—the real world of school, work, and responsibility. Whether a product of television, or more easily influenced by it than normal children, ADHD children are framed in a continuously vulnerable way. Their household requires a special kind of restructuring in which domesticity carefully filters the simulated experiences of the image-based, modern world. Despite obvious differences in their perspective on the cause of ADHD, these discourses propagate similar mechanisms of discipline designed to be enacted on the body of ADHD children.

Through what I have observed as a sincere commitment to evaluating how their children will be disciplined according to the mandates of the ADHD diagnosis, parents' search for alternative interpretations for ADHD does much to dismantle the popular stereotypes of parents who drug their children as easily as they might give them vitamins. The fact that many of the parents I interviewed sought other ways of interpreting and treating their children's behavior demonstrates the high degree of care that is exercised when dealing with their children's health. Their exploration of alternatives—many of which are described as failures—shows the diligence of parents who want to do right by their children.

Despite their etiological and treatment differences, conventional and alternative discourses overlap within domesticity. It is within the domestic realm, in which such a tremendous potential for behavioral regulation exists and in which clinical skills find their application, that these discourses can be seen in their interplay. Within domesticity, behavior modification meets dietary regulation, medication meets MotivAider, television regulation meets "moment-by-moment" children. Common to the seemingly endless application of all of these is a consistent mechanism of discipline. Domesticity must enter into a kind of contract with the means to rectify the manifestations of ADHD. The elements of this contract begin at the level of discourse (i.e., the clinical modalities that make a disorder like ADHD "possible"), which makes its way into popular renditions (i.e., guidebooks and forms of lay commentary), ultimately investing itself in the domestic sphere.

Notes

1. Other than regarding such a position as a "myth," Conners's study does not elaborate why such a criticism of MBD is unfounded.

2. Smith's (1990) position, which urges the critical examination of texts, I believe, runs parallel to Foucault's assertions about the "extradiscursive" dependency, in which social practices are depicted as greatly connected to discursive establishments, or "regimes of truth" (see Barrett 1991, 129). For Foucault, these "regimes" were visible through their institutional manifestations (mental institutions, prisons, schools, hospitals, and so on). It may be argued that Smith's assertions represent a "textual application" of Foucault.

3. Michel Foucault interrogates similar disciplinary modalities in *Discipline and Punish* (1977).

4. In discussing how stigmatized individuals make efforts to mitigate their deviant identity, Goffman (1963) mentions that people suffering from a stigma—and I would also include those who own a "courtesy stigma"—may strive to become experts on the topic of their deviance. For example, recovering drug addicts may become experts on the myths and facts about addiction, and in disseminating this information to others, they transform or reduce their deviant status. In adopting a role as an expert, the stigmatized own responsibility for awareness in the greater community. From Goffman's (1963) perspective, such expertise lessens a stigma's social effects and helps to reconstruct the stigmatized identity into one that is more socially acceptable.

5. A considerable amount of research explores the linkage between ADHD symptoms and diet (Chernick 1980; Forness et al. 1997; Grossman 1982; Janssen et al. 1996; Lindsey and Frith 1982; Mattes 1983; Rowe 1988; Wender 1986; Wolraich 1998). Clinical research on hyperactive children has given the diet hypothesis mixed reviews. For example, a study by Wolraich (1998) concluded that dietary interventions in the daily lives of hyperactive children proved to be inconsequential, prompting either a refutation of the diet hypothesis or a case for considerable reconceptualization of the theory. On the other hand, a study by Rowe (1988) concluded that of fifty-five hyperactive children subjected to a six-week trial of dietary intervention, forty (72 percent) showed marked behavioral improvement.

Chapter Nine

Conclusion

In reflecting upon the contributions of this book and its implications for future social studies of mental health, it is necessary to situate the findings presented here within the greater culture that influences the prevalence and interpretation of ADHD. It is important to examine the ways in which the conditions of modern life affect our perceptions of mental health and the extent to which these perceptions demarcate who is competent, who will succeed, and who will fail. If we were to understand this "cultural idea" of ADHD as directly dependent upon modern societal conditions, the work of Richard DeGrandpre (1999) serves as a good example.

In *Ritalin Nation* (1999), DeGrandpre claims that the prevalence of ADHD results from the conditions of modernity and that the large numbers of children who are today diagnosed with "symptoms" of impulsivity and distractiveness result from a contradictory existence: as a society we are forced into intensified "on-task" behavior in work and school, and simultaneously, with an addict-like willingness, we crave and ingest the Technicolor onslaught of modern society's digitized, shifting, and distracting images. ADHD, according to DeGrandpre, is a product of a social environment that defines success as having the ability to gracefully respond to markedly contradictory demands. To internalize and regard as a kind of reality rapidly shifting media images, and to be able to separate these virtual experiences from the actual world, is to be successful. ADHD, according to this argument, is a moniker for those who lack this success, that is, ADHD summarizes the failure to adapt to the confusing circumstances of modern society. Moreover, Ritalin, the perennial treatment for ADHD, serves as a great equalizer, consumed *en masse* by a society that fails to see its own role in creating the conditions for ADHD.

According to DeGrandpre, rather than addressing the human costs of what he terms "rapid fire culture," our culture engages in a kind of self-serving groupthink in which we pat ourselves on the back for discovering ADHD and regard the discussion of the disorder as one among many in modern medicine. Instead of looking at contemporary culture as potentially harmful to children and adults alike, we take solace in modern psychiatry and its ability to continuously elucidate those mental aberrations that impede productivity and lower one's quality of life. Rapid fire culture fails to ponder ADHD in any critical way because it lacks the time.

DeGrandpre's and others' writings of this ilk, many of which have been addressed in this book, define ADHD as a cultural problem cast in myriad ways. For example, the prevalence of ADHD is exacerbated by parents who are so wrapped up in the demands of modern life that they decide it is easier to diagnose and drug their children than to deal with their children's deeper emotional and intellectual needs. At other moments it is argued that ADHD reflects the state of public education, in which bloated classrooms and stressed-out teachers foster intolerance toward children who cannot sit still. The prevalence of ADHD is also believed to reflect medical practices that equate children to mechanical devices that are easily fixed through appropriate chemical intervention. With these and many other perspectives on the nature of ADHD, an accusing finger is pointed: rapid fire culture may succeed in entertaining children—it successfully gets them in front of the TV until mom and dad come home from work—but it fails to care for them. For children who cannot successfully negotiate the experience of rapid fire culture, the care they receive is pharmacological.

If DeGrandpre and others are correct, we are forced to make the assumption that modernity has won the great battle against the nuances of humanity—that the cookie-cutter mandates of rapid fire culture have succeeded in quashing those subversions and incredulity toward authority that characterize creativity and independence of thought. Despite DeGrandpre's assertions, the participants in this study illustrate that ADHD is a socially negotiated phenomenon. As this book documents, ADHD is riddled with reliability and validity problems, shown in the plurality of ways ADHD is understood. My contention is that there is not one modality that manufactures ADHD for its own convenience, but rather, ADHD is experienced from a variety of personal and professional perspectives that are influenced by myriad factors, including personal evaluation, skepticism, acceptance, and ambivalence. Despite the high prevalence of Ritalin prescriptions in North America and the explosion in ADHD diagnoses in recent years, the everyday experiences surrounding ADHD, as represented by those most closely associated with the disorder, are far from uniform.

Discourse and Group Identity

Even though the experience of ADHD is heterogeneous, it is important not to write-off ADHD as an entirely relativistic, subjective phenomenon. Of primary importance here is the elucidation of what constitutes different forms of group membership in relation to ADHD, something that chapters 3 through 8 of this book have endeavored to illustrate. Despite variation in their perspectives on ADHD, the interviews demonstrate that the consistency in the initial "ADHD encounter" reveals the common thread among group members. For example, clinicians mostly encounter a case of ADHD within the clinical setting—a location that speaks volumes about how ADHD is framed: ADHD is an aberration, framed either as a bona fide illness, a psychodynamic entity, or a combination of the two, and requires medical intervention. Through consistently encountering ADHD within the classroom, teachers also have a unified frame for the disorder: ADHD is an impediment to learning and must be removed in order for the teaching process to be effective. Parents' introduction to ADHD, on the other hand, is specific not to a place but to those with whom parents first discuss the suspicions of their child's having the disorder. Overwhelmingly, these initial suspecting parties are educators, sometimes approaching parents in an individual capacity, sometimes as members of a school-based team. Parents begin to know ADHD, not by the behavior of their children alone, but in how school representatives evaluate the success of their children within that institution. What unifies parents as a respondent group, therefore, is that they initially experience ADHD through their interactions with professionals who explain to them the abnormality of their children's behavior and how such behavior constitutes a significant barrier to present and future success. From these initial and alarming interactions, parents begin the process of acquiring knowledge about ADHD and develop relations with professionals whose job is to treat the disorder.

Interviewing these groups heightens an understanding of how each has a defining experience in negotiating the meanings inherent in ADHD discourse, makes the decision to accept or reject these discourses, and puts its beliefs about ADHD into practice. Through the way beliefs about ADHD make their way into these practices and into the accounts of respondents, we see the staying power of a discourse. The historical and present discussion of stimulant medications, the tenets of neurological and psychodynamic perspectives on ADHD, the arguments that link ADHD to diet—the salience of these and numerous other discussions addressed in this book illustrate this staying power. Borrowing Laclau and Mouffe's (1985) concept of "nodal points" of meaning, the plurality of ADHD perspectives demonstrates that the dominance of one stance toward ADHD is momentary. A nodal point represents the politics of discourse and becomes visible when one discussion has won a sort of ideological battle. Because discourses come and go and the ontologies that they describe may be disregarded at any stage, what has meaning today may be hogwash tomorrow. As they are dependent upon discourse, nodal points are always temporary. Interview data from these respondent groups reflect the momentary nature of meaning, and demonstrate how contradictory perspectives on ADHD can coexist.

Through its seemingly meticulous analysis of data, its medical nomenclature, and its appeal to arguments that invoke the general principles of Western science, neurology has dominated the ADHD discussion in journal articles and technical manuals. But within the realm of social practice, neurology is often fractured hybridized with other perspectives. This calls forth Foucault's theoretical position about the "extradiscursive dependency," which describes how discourses are utilized by people and shape their world view. The extradiscursive dependency reveals human agency. Though a discourse may be dominant, even constituting what Foucault would call a "knowledge regime," the finitudes of how that discourse is applied speak volumes about how humans direct their own lives. Numerous examples of this agency have been seen in the interviews presented here: parents who define their children as "ADHD gifted," teachers who contend that ADHD is gendered because of the structure of the school, clinicians who harbor major reservations about stimulant medications, and so on. Membership in a group, therefore, denotes similarity, not uniformity, in experience.

Supplementing the Sociology of Mental Health: Toward a Synthetic Methodology

Some of the predominant perspectives in the sociology of mental health are valuable in raising awareness of mental disorders, including ADHD. It has been substantiated, for example, that a degree of collusion between labeling agents has occurred throughout the history of ADHD; that the legitimacy of ADHD demonstrates asymmetry between experts and non-experts; and that ADHD experts contribute ideas that become established aspects of dealing with the disorder. The analysis of such dynamics is an established and necessary part of socially exploring mental disorders; a larger discursive-historical purview furthers this critical examination.

Through combining genealogical analyses with interview-based accounts of the social actors surrounding ADHD, this study demonstrates a synthetic approach to the study of mental disorder. Genealogical analyses can be criticized as irrelevant, swimming aimlessly in the value-neutral world of texts. However, when combined with an empirical component, the analysis of discourse can be very fruitful. The everyday conditions of ADHD can be linked to the past and present discussions of the disorder. ADHD, as experienced by lay actors, can be placed within a context that is more encompassing than that of the Goffmanesque "informal/formal" dichotomy. Conversely, the discourse that has comprised the knowledge of ADHD can be seen as an influential factor in the everyday manifestations of the ADHD phenomenon. Both discourse and everyday experience may be analyzed in their reciprocity rather than in their separation from each other. Acknowledging the reciprocity between discourse and everyday experience opens up exciting possibilities for the social study of mental illness.

The use of historical and contemporary frames for ADHD children represents another point at which the sociology of mental health can be expanded to include a more contiguous set of ideas. For example, ADHD suspicions that characterize the relationship between parents and school representatives open the informal/formal dichotomy to more detailed analyses. As they are "semiformal" in how they suspect ADHD children, the clinical capacity with which teachers may operate reveals how a litany of ADHD discussions cultivates expertise, depending upon the professional and personal motivations for attaining that expertise. Furthermore, parents' accumulation of ADHD information demonstrates how established knowledge makes its way into and "formalizes" the informal world. The accessibility of discourse makes the stark distinctions between formal and informal, expert and nonexpert, highly problematic.

This study begins an empirical analysis of discourses effect upon everyday perceptions and, in the context of mental illness, opens up a place for a much larger analysis. As both the legitimacy of knowledge and its points of origin have become increasingly suspect and viewed as political, it is important to examine the way knowledge makes its way into professional and lay consciousness. This would imply an extension of this study's application of interviewing procedures that solicit social actors' relationship to many different and often conflicting bodies of knowledge.

ADHD children become "known" through subscription to information that is framed as legitimate. Formulating the problem of this legitimacy would be a suitable place to begin an empirical analysis of the circulation of knowledge. The establishment of knowledge as legitimate may reveal much about how "good" knowledge is distinguished from "bad." What would need further scrutiny in this regard is how the subscription to particular knowledge reveals the power difference between social actors and those who disseminate it and also how people who previously did not have knowledge about ADHD substantiate themselves as resources of knowledge. An example of this may include a larger analysis of how parents establish themselves as holders of valuable information for others (hence, revealing a reduction in the power asymmetry between themselves and the sources from which they initially learned about ADHD), how clinicians accumulate knowledge and find themselves moving into the "ADHD specialty," and how teachers may solidify a role as a hybrid between clinician and pedagogue.

The findings presented in this book point to research possibilities that can illuminate the largely unexplored social dynamics surrounding ADHD diagnosis and treatment. Outlining the manner in which this mental disorder is negotiated through processes of suspicion and treatment adds a dimension to the study of ADHD that takes into account the attitudes of social actors, their sources of information, and how the allegiance to particular ADHD discourses influences diagnostic and treatment outcomes. ADHD discourse provides a necessary context for the everyday explorations of the disorder. ADHD symptoms have been and continue to be subject to multiple interpretations. Such a condition in the discussions about ADHD extends into and formulates the everyday accounts provided by lay persons. Respondents reveal a multitude of perceptions of the disorder, often leaning toward a neurological perspective on ADHD, but, in a significant number of instances, embracing psychodynamic or combined approaches to the phenomenon. This clearly demonstrates that ADHD is not as cut and dried as many social critics may insist. Instead, ADHD may be seen as a product of a social environment that is characterized by actors with varying relationships to ADHD discourse. Analyzing the relationship between the concepts of mental illnesses as they are represented by books, journal articles, and the like, and the social actors caught in the throes of such illnesses, holds considerable promise for the study of how these phenomena are actuated.

Bibliography

Abrahamson, Isador. "The Epidemic of Lethargic Encephalitis." *New York Medical Record* Dec 11, 1920a.

———. "The Chronicity of Lethargic Encephalitis." *Archives of Neurology and Psychiatry* 4, (1920b): 428-32.

Alexander-Roberts, Colleen. *ADHD and Teens: Proven Techniques for Handling Emotional, Academic and Behavioral Problems.* Dallas: Taylor, 1995.

American Psychiatric Association (APA). APA. *Diagnostic and Statistical Manual of Mental Disorders,* second edition. Washington DC: the Author, 1968.

———. *Diagnostic and Statistical Manual of Mental Disorders,* third edition. Washington DC: the Author, 1980

———. *Diagnostic and Statistical Manual of Mental Disorders,* third edition, revised. Washington DC: the Author, 1987.

———. *Diagnostic and Statistical Manual,* fourth edition. Washington, D.C.: Published by the APA, 1994.

Armstrong, Thomas. *The Myth of the ADD Child.* New York: Plume, 1995.

Arnold, L. Eugene. "ADHD Sex Differences." *Journal of Abnormal Child Psychology* 23, (1995): 555-69.

———. "Sex Differences in ADHD: Conference Summary." *Journal of Abnormal Child Psychology* 23, (1996): 555-69.

———. "NIMH Collaborative Multimodal Treatment Study of Children with Attention-Deficit-Hyperactivity Disorder (MTA)." *Journal of the American Academy of Child and Adolescent Psychiatry* 34 (1997): 987-1000.

Barkley, Russel A. *Attention Deficit Hyperactivity Disorder: A Handbook for Diagnosis and Treatment.* New York: Guilford Press, 1990.

———. *Attention Deficit Hyperactivity Disorder: A Clinical Workbook.* New York: Guilford Press, 1991.

———. "Q: Are Behavior-Modifying Drugs Overprescribed for America's Schoolchildren?" *Insight on the News* 11, no. 31 (1995a): 18-22.

———. *Taking Charge of ADHD: The Complete, Authoritative Guide for Parents.* New York: Guilford, 1995b.

———. *ADHD and the Nature of Self-Control.* London: the Guilford Press, 1997.

Barrett, Michèle. *The Politics of Truth: From Marx to Foucault.* Stanford, CA: Stanford University Press, 1991.

Baving, Lioba, Manfred Laucht, and Martin H. Schmidt. "Atypical Frontal Brain Activation in ADHD: Preschool and Elementary School Boys and Girls." *Journal of the American Academy of Child and Adolescent Psychiatry* 38, (1999): 1363-77.

Becker, Howard S. 1963. *Outsiders: Studies in the Sociology of Deviance.* New York: Free Press.

————. "Interviewing Medical Students." *American Journal of Sociology* 62 (1956): 199-201.

Bender, Lauretta. "Psychological Problems of Children with Organic Brain Disease." *American Journal of Orthopsychiatry* 19 (1949): 404-15.

Bernacki, Peter M. and Dan Waldorf. "Snowball Sampling." *Sociological Methods and Research* 10 (1981): 141-63.

Biederman, Joseph, Stephen Faraone, Erik Mick, Sarah Williamson, Timothy E. Wilens, Thomas J. Spencer, Wendy Weber, Jennifer Jetton, Jim Pert, and Barry Zallen. "Clinical Correlates of ADHD in Females: Findings from a Large Group of Girls Ascertained from Pediatric and Psychiatric Referral Sources." *Journal of the American Academy of Child and Adolescent Psychiatry* 38 (1999): 966-79.

Black, Susan. "Kids Who Can't Sit Still." *Executive Educator* 14 (1992): 31-34.

Bloomingdale, Lewis M. *Attention Deficit Disorder: Diagnostic, Cognitive, and Therapeutic Understanding*. New York: SD Medical and Scientific Books, 1985.

Blum, Allan F. "The Sociology of Mental Illness." In Jack Douglas (ed.), *Deviance and Respectability: The Social Construction of Moral Meanings*. New York: Basic Books, 1970, 31-60.

Blum, Fred H. "Getting Individuals to Give Information to the Outsider." *Journal of Social Issues* 8 (1952): 35-42.

Blumer, Herbert. *Symbolic Interactionism: Perspective and Method*. Berkeley, CA: Univ. of California Press, 1969.

Bradley, Charles. "The Behavior of Children Receiving Benzedrine." *American Journal of Psychiatry* 94 (1937): 577-85.

————. "Benzedrine and Dexedrine in the Treatment of Children's Behavior Disorders." *Pediatrics* 5 (1950): 24-37.

Bradley, Charles, and Margaret Bowen. "School Performance of Children Receiving Amphetamine (Benzedrine) Sulfate." *American Journal of Orthopsychiatry* 10 (1940): 782.

————. "Amphetamine Therapy of Children's Behavior Disorders." *American Journal of Orthopsychiatry* 11 (1941): 92.

Bradley, Charles, and E. Green. "Psychometric Performances of Children Receiving Amphetamine (Benzedrine) Sulfate." *American Journal of Psychiatry* 97 (1940): 388-92.

Bray, Patrick F. *Neurology in Pediatrics*. Chicago: Year Book Medical Publishers, 1969.

Breggin, Peter. "Q: Are Behavior Modifying Drugs being Overprescribed for America's Schoolchildren?" *Insight on the News* 11, no. 31 (1995): 18-22.

————. *Talking Back to Ritalin*. Monroe, ME: Common Courage Press, 1998.

Brewer, John. "Flow of Communications, Expert Qualifications, and Organizational Authority Structures." *American Sociological Review* 36 (1971): 475-84.

Brink, Susan. "Doing Ritalin Right." *U.S. News and World Report* Nov. 23, 1998: 76-81.

Bruno, James E. "Doing Time—Killing Time at School: An Examination of the Perceptions and Allocations of Time Among Teacher-Defined At-Risk Students." *Urban Review* 27 (1995): 101-20.

Buchoff, Rita. "Attention Deficit Disorder: Help for the Classroom Teacher." *Childhood Education* 67 (1990): 86-90.

Burnley, Georgia. "A Team Approach for Identification of Attention Deficit Hyperactivity Disorder." *School Counselor* 40 (1993): 228-30.

Cantwell, Dennis P. "Foreward." In Russell Barkley, *Hyperactive Children: A Handbook for Diagnosis and Treatment.* New York: Guilford, 1981, vii-x.

Carroll, William K. and Robert S. Ratner. "Master-Framing and Cross-Movement Networking in Contemporary Social Movements." *The Sociological Quarterly 37* (1996): 601-25.

Chase, Marilyn. "Studies of Ritalin's Role in Drug Abuse Produce Contradictory Findings." *Wall Street Journal* 233, no. 95 (1999): B1.

Chernick, Eleanor. "Effects of the Feingold Diet on Reading Achievement and Classroom Behavior." *Reading Teacher* 34, (1980): 171-3.

Connell, Philip H. *Amphetamine Psychosis.* London: Chapman and Hall, 1958.

Conners, C. Keith. "Psychological Effects of Stimulant Drugs in Children with Minimal Brain Dysfunction." *Pediatrics* 49 (1972): 702-8.

Conners, C. Keith, and Leon Eisenberg. "The Effects of Methylphenidate on Symptomatology and Learning in Disturbed Children." *American Journal of Psychiatry* 12, (1963): 458-64.

Conrad, Peter. "The Discovery of Hyperkinesis: Notes on the Medicalization of Deviant Behavior." *Social Problems* 23 (1975): 12-21.

———. *Identifying Hyperactive Children: The Medicalization of Deviant Behavior.* Lexington, MA: Lexington Books, 1976.

Conrad, Peter and Deborah Potter. "From Hyperactive Children to ADHD Adults: Observations on the Expansion of Medical Categories." *Social Problems* 47 (2000): 559-82.

Conrad, Peter and Joseph Schneider. *Deviance and Medicalization: From Badness to Sickness.* St. Louis: Mosby, 1980.

Cruikshank, Julie. *The Social Life of Stories: Narrative and Knowledge in the Yukon Territory.* Lincoln, NB: Univ. of Nebraska Press, 1998.

DeGrandpre, Richard. *Ritalin Nation: Rapid-Fire Culture and the Transformation of Human Consciousness.* New York: W.W. Norton, 1999.

Denzin, Norman K. *Interpretive Interactionism.* London: Sage, 1989.

———. "The Practices of Politics on Interpretation." In Norman Denzin and Yvonne Lincoln (eds.), *Handbook of Qualitative Research.* Thousand Oaks, CA: Sage, 2000, 897-922.

Diller, Lawrence H. *Running on Ritalin: A Physician Reflects on Children, Society, and Performance in a Pill.* New York: Bantam Books, 1998.

Dorman, Steven M. "Video and Computer Games: Effect on Children and Implications for Health. *Journal of School Health* 67 (1997): 133-8.

Douglas, Jack D. *Deviance and Respectability: The Social Construction of Moral Meanings.* Basic Books: New York, 1970.

Douglas, Virginia I., Gabrielle Weiss, and Mindie Klauss. "Learning Disabilities in Hyperactive Children and the Effects of Methylphenidate." *Canadian Psychologist* 10 (1969): 201.

Dowdy, Carol A. *Attention Deficit/Hyperactivity Disorder in the Classroom: A Practical Guide for Teachers*. Austin, TX: Pro-Ed, 1998.

Dumont, Matthew. "Focusing on Television." *American Journal of Psychiatry* 133 (1976): 457.

Dyer-Wiley, Collen M. "Dealing with a Disruptive Child." *Principal* 78 (1999): 30-1.

Ebaugh, Franklin G. "Neuropsychiatric Sequelae of Acute Epidemic Encephalitis in Children." *American Journal of Diseases of Children* 25 (1923): 89-97.

Eisenberg, Leon. "The Clinical Use of Stimulant Drugs in Children." *Pediatrics* 49 (1972): 709-15.

Eisenberg, Leon, Roy Lachman, Peter E. Molling, Arthur Lockner, James D Mizelle, and C. Keith Conners. "A Psychopharmacologic Experiment in a Training School for Delinquent Boys." *American Journal of Orthopsychiatry* 33 (1963): 431.

Emerson, Robert M., and Sheldon L. Messinger. "The Micro-Politics of Trouble." *Social Problems* 25 (1977): 121-34.

Feingold, Ben F. *Why Your Child Is Hyperactive*. New York: Random House, 1974.

Flick, Grad L. *Power Parenting for Children with ADD/ADHD:A Practical Parent's Guide for Managing Difficult Behavior*. New York: Simon and Schuster, 1996.

Fontana, Andrea, and James H. Frey. "The Interview: From Structured Questions to Negotiated Text." In Norman Denzin and Yvonne Lincoln (eds.), *Handbook of Qualitative Research*. Thousand Oaks, CA: Sage, 2000, 361-76.

Ford, Frank R. *Diseases of the Nervous System in Infancy, Childhood, and Adolescence*. Springfield, Ill: Charles C. Thomas, 1948.

Forness, Steven R., Kenneth A. Kavale, Ilaina M. Blum, and John W. Lloyd. "Mega-Analysis of Meta-Analyses: What Works in Special Education and Related Services." *Teaching Exceptional Children* 29 (1997): 4-9.

Foucault, Michel. *Madness and Civilization: A History of Insanity in the Age of Reason*. New York: Random House, 1965.

———. *The Birth of the Clinic: An Archaeology of Medical Perception*. New York: Vintage, 1973.

———. *Discipline and Punish: the Birth of the Prison*. New York: Pantheon, 1977.

———. "Politics and Study of Discourse." *Ideology and Consciousness* 3 (1978): 7-26.

Fraser, Nancy. *Unruly Practices: Power, Discourse, and Gender in Contemporary Social Theory*. Minneapolis: University of Minnesota Press, 1989.

Freud, Anna. *Psycho-Analytical Treatment of Children: Technical Lectures and Essays by Anna Freud*. New York: International Universities Press, 1926.

Fuster, Joaquin M. *The Prefrontal Cortex: Anatomy, Physiology, and Neuropsychology of the Frontal Lobe*. New York: Raven, 1997.

Gadow, Kenneth D. *Children on Medication*. San Diego, CA: College Hill Press, 1986.

Gaub, Miranda, and Caryn L. Carlson. "Gender Differences in ADHD: A Meta-Analysis and Critical Review." *Journal of the American Academy of Child and Adolescent Psychiatry* 36 (1997): 1036-46.

Glaser, Barney G. *Theoretical Sensitivity: Advances in the Methodology of Grounded Theory*. Mill Valley, CA: The Sociology Press, 1978.

Glaser, Barney G. and Anselm L. Strauss. *The Discovery of Grounded Theory: Strategies for Qualitative Research*. Chicago: Aldine, 1967.

Goddard, Henry H. *The Criminal Imbecile*. New York: MacMillan, 1915.

Goffman, Erving. *The Presentation of Self in Everyday life*. New York: Anchor, 1959.

———. *Asylums: Notes on the Social Situation of Mental Patients and Other Inmates*. New York: Anchor, 1961.

———. *Stigma: Notes on the Management of Spoiled Identity*. New York: Touchstone, 1963.

———. *Behavior in Public Place*: Notes on the Social Organization of Gatherings. New York: The Free Press, 1964.

Goldman, Larry S., Myron Genel., Rebecca J. Bezman, and Priscilla J. Slanetz, for the Council on Scientific Affairs, American Medical Association. "Diagnosis and Treatment of Attention-Deficit/Hyperactivity Disorder in Children and Adolescents." *Journal of the American Medical Association* 279 (1998): 1100-07.

Greenacre, Phyllis. "The Predisposition to Anxiety." *Psychoanalytic Quarterly* 10 (1941): 66-94.

Greene, Ross W. "Students with Attention Deficit Hyperactivity Disorder in School Classrooms: Teacher Factors Related to Compatibility, Assessment and Intervention." *School Psychology Review* 24 (1995): 81-93.

Greenhill, Laurence L. "Medication Treatment Strategies in the MTA: Relevance to Clinicians and Researchers." *Journal of the American Academy of Child and Adolescent Psychiatry* 35 (1996): 1304-13.

Grossman, Eugene. "The Feingold Diet for the Hyperactive Child." *American Family Physician* 26 (1982): 101-2.

Grusky, Oscar, and Melvin Pollner (eds.) *The Sociology of Mental Illness: Basic Studies*. New York: Reinhart, 1981.

Habermas, Jürgen. *The Philosophical Discourse of Modernity: Twelve Lectures*. Cambridge: MIT Press, 1984.

Hacking, Ian. *Rewriting the Soul*. Princeton: Princeton University Press, 1995.

Hallowell, Edward M. and John J. Ratey. *Driven to Distraction: Recognizing and Coping with Attention Deficit Disorder from Childhood through Adulthood*. New York: Touchstone, 1994.

Hohman, Leslie B. "Postencephalitic Behavior Disorders in Children." *Johns Hopkins Hospital Bulletin* 33 (1922): 372-5.

Ireland, William W. *On Idiocy and Imbecility.* London: J & A Churchill, 1877.

———. *The Mental Affectations of Idiocy, Imbecility and Insanity.* Philadelphia: P. Blakiston's, 1900.

Jacobs, Edward H. *Fathering the ADHD Child: A Book for Fathers, Mothers, and Professionals.* New York: Jason Aronson, 1998.

Janssen, Karin, Peter Hollman, Dini P. Venema, Wija van Staveren, and Martijn B. Katan. "Salicylates in Food." *NutritionReview* 54 (1996): 357-60.

Jensen, Martin D., and Dennis P. Cantwell. "Comorbidity in ADHD: Implications to Research, Practice and DSM IV. *Journal of the American Academy of Child and Adolescent Psychiatry* 36 (1997): 1065-79.

Jordan, Dale R. *Attention Deficit Disorder: The ADD Syndrome.* Austin, TX: Pro-Ed, 1988.

Karp, David. "Illness Ambiguity and the Search for Meaning: A Case Study of a Self-Help Group for Affective Disorders." *Journal of Contemporary Ethnography* 21 (1992): 139-170.

———. *Speaking of Sadness: Illness, Identity, and the Meaning of Disconnection.* New York: Oxford, 1996.

Keepers, George A. "Pathological Preoccupation with Video Games." *Journal of the American Academy of Child and Adolescent Psychiatry* 29 (1990): 49-50.

Kennedy, Roger L. J. "The Prognosis of Sequelae of Epidemic Encephalitis in Children." *American Journal of Diseases of Children* 28 (1924): 158-172.

Kessler, Jane W. "History of Minimal Brain Dysfunctions." in Herbert and Ellen Rie (eds.) *Handbook of Minimal Brain Dysfunction: A Critical View.* New York: Wiley-Interscience, 1980, 18-42.

Kirk, Stuart A. and Herb Kutchins. *The Selling of DSM: The Rhetoric of Science in Psychiatry.* Chicago: Aldine, 1992.

Kivett, Douglas D. and Carol A.B. Warren. "Social Control in a Group Home for Delinquent Boys." *Journal of Contemporary Ethnography* 31 (2002): 3-33.

Klein, Melanie. *The Psychoanalysis of Children.* London: The Hogarth Press Ltd., 1963 (originally published as *Die Psychoanalyse des Kindes,* 1932).

Kramer, Peter. *Listening to Prozac: A Psychiatrist Explores Antidepressant Drugs and the Remaking of the Self.* New York: Penguin, 1993.

Laclau, Ernesto, and Chantal Mouffe. *Hegemony and Socialist Strategy: Towards a Radical Democratic Politics.* London: Verso, 1985.

Lemert, Edwin. "Paranoia and the Dynamics of Exclusion." *Sociometry* 25 (1962): 2-20.

Lindsey, Jimmy D., and Greg H. Frith. "Hyperkinesis, Nutrition, and the Feingold Diet: Implications for Rehabilitation Specialists." *Journal of Rehabilitation* 48 (1982): 69-71.

Lombroso, Cesare. *L'Uomo Delinquente.* Bocca: Turin, 1876.

Lucas, Alexander R., and Morris Weiss. "Methylphenidate Hallucinosis." *Journal of the American Medical Association* 217 (1971): 1079-81.

Marks, Alexandra. "Schoolyard Hustlers' New Drug: Ritalin." *Christian Science Monitor* 92, no. 237 (2000): 1.

Marshall, Gordon. *The Concise Oxford Dictionary of Sociology.* Oxford: Oxford Press, 1996.

Mataro, Maria. "Magnetic Resonance Imaging Measurement of the Caudate Nucleus in Adolescents with Attention Deficit-Hyperactivity Disorder and its Relationship with Neuropsychological and Behavioral Measures." *Archives of Neurology* 54, (1997): 963-8.

Mate, Gabor. *Scattered Minds: A New Look at the Origins and Healing of Attention Deficit Disorder.* Toronto: Vintage Canada, 2000.

Matthys, Walter, Juliane M. Cuperus, and Herman van Engeland. "Deficient Social Problem-Solving in Boys with ODD/CD, with ADHD and with Both Disorders." *Journal of the American Academy of Child and Adolescent Psychiatry* 38 (1999): 311-25.

Mattes, Jeffrey A. "The Feingold Diet: A Current Reappraisal." *Journal of Learning Disabilities* 16 (1983): 319-23.

Maynard, Douglas W. "Language, Interaction, and Social Problems." *Social Problems* 35 (1988): 311-34.

McCall, Robert B. "ADD Alert!" *Learning* 17 (1989): 66-9.

McFarland, Dianna L., Rosemarie Kolstad, and L.D. Briggs. "Educating Attention Deficit-Hyperactivity Disorder Children. *Education* 115 (1995): 595-603.

McKegany, Neil. "No Doubt She's Really a Little Princess: A Case Study of Trouble in a Therapeutic Community." *Sociological Review* 32 (1984): 328-49.

Mercier, Charles A. *Sanity and Insanity.* London: Scott, 1890.

———. "Moral Imbecility." *Practitioner.* October (1917): 301-8.

Meyer, Marshall L. "Experts and the Span of Control." *American Sociological Review* 33 (1968): 944-51.

Miller, Gale. "Holding Clients Accountable: The Micro-Politics of Trouble in a Work Incentive Program." *Social Problems* 31 (1983): 139-52.

Miller, Gale, and David Silverman. "Troubles Talk and Counseling Discourse: A Comparative Study." *The Sociological Quarterly* 36 (1995): 725-47.

Moore, Thomas J. *Prescription for Disaster.* New York: Simon and Schuster, 1998.

Motlitch, Matthew, and August K. Eccles. "Effect of Benzedrine Sulfate on Intelligence Scores of Children." *American Journal of Psychiatry* 94 (1937): 587-90.

Motlitch, Matthew and John P. Sullivan. "Effect of Benzedrine Sulfate on Children taking the new Stanford Achievement Test." *American Journal of Orthopsychiatry* 7 (1937): 519-22.

Ney, Philip G. "Psychosis in a Child Associated with Amphetamine Administration." *Canadian Medical Association Journal* 97, (1967): 1026-8.

Nicholls, Tracey. "A Paradoxical Effect: Across the Continent, Young Killers Prove to be Graduates of Ritalin Therapy." *News Magazine* 23 (August 1999): 22.

Nicklin, Julie L. "The Latest Trend: Mixing Prescription Drugs with Other Stimulants." *Chronicle of Higher Education* 46, no. 40 (2000): A58.

Paterson, Donald, and John C. Spence. "The After-Effects of Epidemic Encephalitis in Children." *The Lancet* (September 3, 1921): 491-3.

Pfiffner, Linda J. *All about ADHD: The Complete Practical Guide for Classroom Teachers.* New York: Scholastic Professional Books, 1996.

Power, Thomas, and George J. DuPaul. "Implications of *DSM IV* for the Practice of School Psychology." *School Psychology Review* 25 (1996): 55-58.

Rank, Beata. "Intensive Study and Treatment of Preschool Children who Show Marked Personality Deviations or 'Atypical Development' and their Parents." Paper presented to International Institute of Child Psychiatry, Toronto, August, 1954.

Reason, Rea. "ADHD: A Psychological Response to an Evolving Concept." *Journal of Learning Disabilities* 32 (1999): 85-101.

Richters, John E. "NIMH Collaborative Multi-Modal Treatment Study of Children with Attention Deficit-Hyperactivity Disorder." *Journal of the American Academy of Child and Adolescent Psychiatry* 54, (1997): 865-70.

Rosenhan, David L. "Being Sane in Insane Places." *Science* 179, (1973): 250-8.

Rowe, Katherine S. "Synthetic Food Colourings and 'Hyperactivity': A Double-Blind Crossover Study." *Australian Paediatric Journal* 24 (1988): 143-7.

Rutstein, Nat. *"Go Watch TV!": What and How Much Should Children Really Watch?* New York: Sheid and Ward, 1974.

Scheff, Thomas. *Being Mentally Ill: A Sociological Theory.* New York: Aldine De Gruyter, 1999.

Schrag, Peter, and Diane Divoky. *The Myth of the Hyperactive Child and Other Means of Child Control.* New York: Pantheon, 1975.

Schultz, Margaret. "WISC-III and WJ-R Tests of Achievement: Concurrent Validity and Learning Disability Identification. *Journal of Special Education* 31 (1997): 377-86.

Sheridan, Susan M., Candace L. Dee, Julie C. Morgan, Megan E. McCormick, and Darlene Walker. "A Multi-Method Intervention for Social Skills Deficits in Children with ADHD and their Parents. *School Psychology Review* 25 (1996): 57-76.

Smith, Dorothy E. *The Conceptual Practices of Power: A Feminist Sociology of Knowledge.* Toronto: University of Toronto Press, 1990.

Sommers, Christina H. *The War Against Boys: How Misguided Feminism is Harming our Young Men.* New York: Touchstone, 2000.

Snow, David A. and Robert D. Benford. "Ideology, Frame Resonance, and Participant Mobilization." *Interactional Social Movement Research* 1 (1988): 197-217.

Soper, William B., and Mark J. Miller. "Junk-Time Junkies: An Emerging Addiction Among Students. *School Counselor* 31 (1983): 40-43.

Stewart, Mark A. "Hyperactive Children." *Scientific American* 222 (1970): 94-98.

Still, George F. "Some Abnormal Psychical Conditions in Children." *The Lancet* (April 12, 19, 26, 1902): 1008-12, 1079-82, 1163-67.

Strauss, Anselm, and Juliet Corbin. *Grounded Theory in Practice*. London: Sage, 1997.

Strecker, Edward A. "Behavior Problems in Encephalitis." *Archives of Neurology and Psychiatry* 21 (1929): 137-44.

Stryker, Sue B. "Encephalitis Lethargica: the Behavior Residuals." *The Training School Bulletin* 22 (1925): 152-7.

Szasz, Thomas. *The Myth of Mental Illness: Foundations of a Theory of Personal Conduct*. New York: Harper Collins, 1974.

Tredgold, Alfred F. "Moral Imbecility." *Practitioner* (July 1917): 43-56.

Trice, Harrison M. "The 'Outsider's' Role in Field Study." *Sociology and Social Research* 41 (1970): 27-32.

Walker, Sidney. *The Hyperactivity Hoax*. New York: St. Martin's Press, 1998.

Webb, Eugene J., Donald T. Campbell, Richard D. Schwartz, and Lee Sechrest. *Unobtrusive Measures: Non-Reactive Research in the Social Sciences*. Chicago: Rand McNally, 1966.

Webster, Stephen, and Richard O'Toole. "Problems in Identifying, Reporting, and Treating Family Mistreatment: Roles for the Applied Sociologist." *Sociological Focus* 22 (1989): 181-190.

Weinberg, Darin. "The Social Construction of Non-Human Agency: The Case of Mental Disorder." *Social Problems* 44 (1997): 217-35.

Weingartner, Paul L. *ADHD Handbook for Families: A Guide to Communicating with Professionals*. Washington, DC: Child and Family Press, 1999.

Wender, Esther H. "The Food Additive-Free Diet in the Treatment of Behavior Disorders: A Review." *Journal of Developmental and Behavioral Paediatrics* 7 (1986): 35-42.

Wender, Paul. *Minimal Brain Dysfunction in Children*. New York: Wiley-Interscience, 1971.

Winn, Marie. *The Plug-in Drug: Television and the Family*. New York: Penguin, 1985.

Wolraich, Mark L. "Comparison of Diagnostic Criteria for ADHD in a County-wide Sample." *Journal of the American Academy of Child and Adolescent Psychiatry* 35 (1996): 319-24.

———. "Attention Deficit Hyperactivity Disorder." *Professional Care of Mother and Child* 8 (1998): 35-37.

Wronski, Richard. "New Screen Gauges Hyperactivity." *Chicago Tribune*. (July 25, 2001): B3.

Young, Allan. *The Harmony of Illusions: Inventing Post-Traumatic Stress Disorder*. Princeton, NJ: Princeton University Press, 1995.

Young, David, and William Beecher Scoville. "Paranoid Psychosis in Narcolepsy and the Possible Danger of Benzedrine Treatment." *Medical Clinics of North America* 22 (1938): 637-46.

Index

Abrahamson, Isador, 29-30
Adderall, 2
aggressive behavior, 144
agnosias, 48
Alexander-Roberts, Colleen, 162
American Academy of Pediatrics, 2
American Psychiatric Association, 15; *Diagnostic and Statistical Manual of Mental Disorders* and the, 35, 44, 50, 117, 131, 132, 139, 166
aphasias, 48
apraxias, 48
Armstrong, Thomas, 39, 171
Arnold, L. Eugene, 8
Attention Deficit Hyperactivity Disorder, 1-3; academic and social struggles in connection to, 131-33; behavioral problems and, 41; diagnosis of, 50; as a disability, 73; as gendered problem, 8, 17, 109; genetic explanations for, 163-64; neurological perspectives on, 43; organic and social causes of, 48; potential overdiagnosis of, 45; psychodynamic perspective on, 43; symptoms of, 1
atypical ego development, 7
autoerotic gratification, 38

Barkley, Russel A., 21, 27, 29, 33, 55, 58, 154, 159, 160, 171
Barrett, Michèle, 10
Baving, Lioba, 60
Becker, Howard S., 4, 12, 129
behavior modification, 156

behavior testing for ADHD, 52
Bender, Lauretta, 39
Bender-Gestalt test, 48
Benzedrine, 70-71, 157
Biederman, Joseph, 8
Biernaki, Peter, 12
Black, Susan, 90
Bloomingdale, Lewis M., 90
Blum, Fred, 12
Blumer, Herbert, 5
Bradley, Charles, 16, 70-71, 73, 81, 88, 157
Bray, Patrick F., 48
Breggin, Peter, 50, 58, 157
Brewer, John, 151
Briggs, L. D., 91
Brink, Susan, 55
British Mental Deficiency Act of 1913, 26
Bruno, James E., 173
Buchoff, Rita, 90
Burnley, Georgia, 103

caffeine, 168
Cantwell, Dennis P., 60
Carroll, William K., 69
Chase, Marilyn, 85
chemical therapy, 40
Chernick, Eleanor, 175
classroom structure for special needs children, 89
clinicians, definition of, 12
compulsion neurosis, 37
conduct disorder, 144
Connell, Philip, 80
Conners, C. Keith, 157-59

Conners Scale, 52-57
Conrad, Peter, 3-5, 49
courtesy stigma, 155
Cruikshank, Julie, 12
Cylert, 2, 89

daydreaming as indication of
    ADHD, 132
defective ego, 38
DeGrandpre, Richard, 172, 177-78
delinquency, 29, 32
dementia naturalis, 23
Denzin, Norman K., 12
deviant behavior, 47, 110, 121, 129
Dexedrine, 2, 166
Diller, Lawrence H., 39, 47
disease process narrative of
    ADHD, 53-57
Divoky, Diane, 21, 90
dopamine disregulation, 55-56;
    Ritalin usage and, 63
Dorman, Steven M., 173
Douglas, Jack D., 5
Douglas, Virginia I., 88
Dowdy, Carol A., 104
Dumont, Matthew, 172-173
DuPaul, George, 91
Dyer-Wiley, Collen M., 91

Ebaugh, Franklin G., 30
Eisenberg, Leon, 49
Emerson, Robert M., 5, 129, 132,
    142-143, 148-149, 152
encephalitis lethargica, 7, 15, 39,
    49, 90; behavior residuals of, 30-
    34; as medical explanation for
    delinquency, 29; motor behaviors
    and, 33; studied behaviors and,
    33

Feingold, Ben F., 168
Feingold diet, 168-70
Fetal Alcohol Syndrome (FAS), 98

fidgetiness, 37
Flick, Grad L., 160, 171
Fontana, Andrea, 12
food, drug, and cosmetic Yellow
    #5, Tartrazine, 169
Ford, Frank R., 48
Forness, Steven R., 175
Foucault, Michel, 8-9, 25, 59, 180
Fraser, Nancy, 11
Freud, Anna, 36, 125, 132
Frey, James H., 12
Fuster, Joaquin M., 55

Gadow, Kenneth D., 90
garbage can diagnosis, 146
Gaub, Miranda, 8
genealogical methods, 7-8, 181
Glaser, Barney G., 12
Goddard, Henry H., 24
Goffman, Erving, 5, 12, 105, 130,
    155, 181
Goldman, Larry S., 78
Greenacre, Phyllis, 38, 53
Greene, Ross W., 91
Greenhill, Laurence L., 73
group identity and orientation to
    ADHD, 179
Grossman, Eugene, 175
Grusky, Oscar, 6

Habermas, Jürgen, 11
Hacking, Ian, 9
Hallowell, Edward M., 161
high intelligence and ADHD, 139
Hohman, Leslie B., 30
homo criminalis, 25
hyperactivity, 34, 51, 117, 131,
    168-169
hyperkinesis, 3, 18, 44

idiocy, 15, 21-23
imbecility, 15, 21-23
impulsivity, 34, 51

inattention, 51
Individual Education Plans (IEPs), 103
infant neuroses, 36
insurance company compensation, 45
internal locus of control, 83-84
International Institute of Child Psychiatry, 38
intervention in classrooms, 110-12
Ireland, William W., 22, 24-25

Jacobs, Edward H., 160
Janssen, Karin, 175
Jensen, Martin D., 60
Jordan, Dale R., 95-96

Karp, David, 19, 130
Keepers, George A., 173
Kennedy, Roger L. J., 30
Kessler, Jane W., 21, 29-30, 33
kinesthetic learners, 94
Kirk, Stuart A., 45, 50
Kivett, Douglas D., 130
Klein, Melanie, 36
Kolstad, Rosemarie, 91
Kutchins, Herb, 45, 50

labeling approaches to ADHD, 119-23
Laclau, Ernesto, 180
learning assistance center, 113
learning disability, 138
Lemert, Edwin, 120
Lindsey, Jimmy D., 175
Lombroso, Cesare, 28
Lucas, Alexander R., 81

Mataro, Maria, 58
Mate, Gabor, 56, 166
Matthys, Walter, 58
Mattes, Jeffrey A., 175
Maynard, Douglas W., 129

McCall, Robert B., 90
McFarland, Dianna L., 91
McKeganey, Neil, 130
medicalization, 2, 17
Mercier, Charles A., 23, 26, 28
Messinger, Sheldon, 5, 129, 131-132, 142-143, 148-149, 152
Meyer, Marshall L., 151
micropolitics of trouble, 142, 152
Miller, Gale, 129-130,
Miller, Mark, 173
minimal brain damage, 7, 49
minimal brain dysfunction, 4, 7, 49
minimal cerebral palsy, 7, 49
Moore, Thomas J., 8
Motiv-Aider device, 155, 174
Motlitch, Matthew, 71
Mouffe, 180
multiple personality disorder, 9

narcissistic gratification, 38
Ney, Philip G., 80
Nicholls, Tracey, 157
Nicklin, Julie L., 85
Nintendo, 171
Novartis Pharmaceuticals, 3

optical tracking and attention test, 58
O'Toole, Richard, 130

Paterson, Donald, 30
Pfiffner, Linda J., 90
Pollner, Melvin, 6
positron emission tomography, 57
postmodern methodology, 10
Post-Traumatic Stress Disorder (PTSD), 9
Power, Thomas, 91
Proctor-Gregg, Nancy, 37
psychopharmacology, 159

Rank, Beata, 38

Ratey, John, 162
Ratner, Robert S., 69
Reason, Rea, 78
residual rule breaking, 6
retardation, 32
Richters, John E., 73
Ritalin, 1-2, 40-43, 57, 76, 89, 117,
    147-148; drug abuse and, 156-
    157; misdiagnosis and, 45; psy-
    choses and, 78-83
Rosenhan, David L., 120
Rowe, Katherine S., 175
Royal College of Physicians, 24
Rutstein, Nat, 173

Scheff, Thomas, 6, 106
Schizophrenia, 10, 54
Schneider, Joseph, 6
school-based team (SBT), 103,
    137, 147
school curricula, 109; assignment
    modification of, 112; interven-
    tion strategies and, 136; social
    deviance and, 110
Schrag, Peter, 21, 90
Schultz, Margaret, 91
secondary diagnoses, 41
self-centeredness, 38
Sheridan, Susan M., 91
Silverman, David, 129
sleepy sickness, 29. *See also en-
    cephalitis lethargica*
Smith, Dorothy E., 160-161
Snow, David A., 69
snowball approach to data collec-
    tion, 12
social determinism, 11
social incompetence, 120
Sommers, Christina H., 126-127
Sontag, Susan, 11
Soper, William B., 173

Stewart, Mark A., 33
Still, George F., 15, 21, 26-27, 145
stimulant medications, 12, 16
Strauss, Anselm, 12
Strecker, Edward A., 33
Stryker, Sue B., 30
Symbolic Interactionism, 5
synthetic methodology in the soci-
    ology of mental health, 180
Szasz, Thomas, 41

Teicher, Martin, 58
television and ADHD symptoms,
    18, 171-172
trauma as cause for ADHD, 39
Tredgold, Alfred F., 26, 28
Trice, Harrison M., 12

United States Public Health Ser-
    vice, 49

video games and ADHD symp-
    toms, 18, 171-172
violent behavior and ADHD, 141

waivering calibrations, 14
Waldorf, Dan, 12
Walker, Sidney, 58
Warren, Carol, 130
Webb, Eugene J., 14
Webster, Stephen, 130
Weinberg, Darin, 99, 164
Weingartner, Paul L., 160
Wender, Esther H., 175
Wender, Paul, 49, 53-54
Winn, Marie, 173
Wolraich, Mark L., 92
Wronski, Richard, 58

Young, Allan, 9
Young, David, 80

About the Author

Adam Rafalovich is assistant professor of sociology at Texas Tech University, where he was recently the recipient of a Professing Excellence Award. He holds a Ph.D. in sociology from the University of British Columbia and has published widely on the topic of ADHD, with articles appearing in *Deviant Behavior*, *The Sociological Quarterly*, and *Journal for the Theory of Social Behaviour*. An avid musician and backpacker, he and his wife Nell live in Lubbock, Texas.